THE ENCYCLOPEDIA OF
HEALING POINTS

The ENCYCLOPEDIA of HEALING POINTS

THE HOME GUIDE TO ACUPOINT TREATMENT

ROGER DALET, M.D.

Translated by Jon E. Graham

Healing Arts Press
Rochester, Vermont • Toronto, Canada

Healing Arts Press
One Park Street
Rochester, Vermont 05767
www.HealingArtsPress.com

Healing Arts Press is a division of Inner Traditions International

Originally published in French under the title *Encyclopédie des points qui guérissent: La santé au bout des doigts* by Éditions Jouvence
First U.S. edition published in 2010 by Healing Arts Press

Note to the reader: *This book is intended as an informational guide. The remedies, approaches, and techniques described herein are meant to supplement, and not to be a substitute for, professional medical care or treatment. They should not be used to treat a serious ailment without prior consultation with a qualified health care professional.*

Library of Congress Cataloging-in-Publication Data
Dalet, Roger.
  [Encyclopédie des points qui guérissent. English]
  The encyclopedia of healing points : the home guide to acupoint treatment / Roger Dalet ; translated by Jon E. Graham. —1st U.S. ed.
      p. cm.
  Summary: "A complete home health guide for treating more than 150 common illnesses with the stimulation of acupoints"—Provided by publisher.
  Includes index.
  ISBN 978-1-59477-335-8 (pbk.)
  1. Acupuncture—Popular works. I. Title.
  RM184.D25513 2010
  615.8'92—dc22
                                                              2010009747

Printed and bound in India by Replika Press Pvt. Ltd.

10   9   8   7   6   5   4   3   2   1

Text design and layout by Virginia Scott Bowman
This book was typeset in Life with Bauer Bodoni and Gill Sans as display typefaces

Contents

Digestion

Circulation

Urinary System

PART ELEVEN

Reproductive Health

PART TWELVE

Miscellaneous

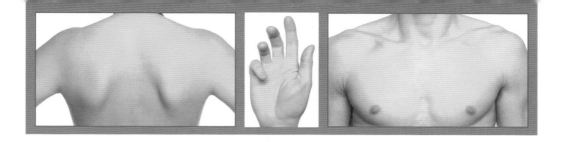

Introduction

THIS BOOK IS directed at both health professionals and individuals seeking to take control of their own health. Some of the techniques are quite convenient for home use, while others—generally those directed at more serious conditions—will require the guidance of a trained practitioner.

I have selected only the most common illnesses and disorders for inclusion, and have arranged this book in a way that should make it easy for the reader to use regularly. Each condition is accompanied by a brief description of its symptoms and the conventional treatment normally applied to them. I then describe for each ailment the acupuncture points that Chinese medicine would commonly recommend for such a condition, and any additional points that I have found to be particularly effective in my own long experience as a practitioner. The points are then divided into principal and secondary points. As a general rule, stimulation of the principal points is enough to provide an active therapeutic effect. The secondary points are used to reinforce or adjust the effects of the primary points.

HOW THE POINTS ARE STIMULATED

While acupuncture with fine stainless steel needles is still the most well-known method of stimulating acupoints, there are many other ways, several of which can be easily accomplished by lay readers. This book focuses on two simple methods that are safe and easy to practice at home.

Simple Manual Massage
Place the tip of your thumb or index finger on the point indicated (this can even be an approximate placement) and lightly vibrate your finger or rotate it clockwise while pressing down sharply. More precise pressure can be applied on a point by using the eraser end of a pencil or a small thimble. Success is obtained when the symptom—the pain or disorder or sick feeling—disappears. For treatment of chronic illnesses you should perform this same massage twice a day for two to ten minutes at a time.

Electrical Stimulation
For many years, researchers have sought to develop alternate ways of stimulating

acupoints. The application of electrical current began in China in the 1930s; today, this effort has been expanded by the advent of newer, simpler, and more reliable machines. Whereas the original devices required that electrodes be attached to needles inserted in the skin—and therefore could only be used by professional acupuncturists—some of the more modern stimulators can be applied directly to the skin, and can thus be used by nonprofessionals.

THE EVOLUTION OF ACUPOINT THERAPY

Acupuncture appears to be the oldest system of medicine on the planet. Its origins are lost in the dawn of time, but archaeological discoveries and subsequent extensive research performed in China show evidence of acupuncture's use more than two thousand years ago. In written works dating from before the birth of Christ, researchers have discovered clear discussions of acupuncture needling.

Acupressure—the stimulation of acupuncture points by hand—may even have predated the use of needles. Without clear written documents, however, it is hard to know exactly how these styles of medicine evolved.

How is it that we have no written documents recording the origins of acupuncture or acupressure? The major reason is the draconian laws established by a Chinese ruler, Emperor Huang-Ti, around 200 BCE. This sovereign ordered all the books existing in China at this time destroyed, because he

wished for no evidence to survive from the time preceding his rule.

On the other hand, he did take pains to see that medical treatises were written. He literally imposed the method of their creation when he wrote: "I desire to put an end to the use of medicines that poison . . . I wish only the mysterious metal needles to be used."

If these needles were a mystery to him, just imagine how much greater their mysteries are for us!

Following the death of this terrible autocrat, those who outlived his reign compared what they remembered of the documents he had destroyed and wrote the first acupuncture "books," primarily the *Nei Jing* and the *Su Wen*. While the instructions in these books sometimes match, they often diverge and even contradict each other. For this reason the contradictory nature of traditional Chinese medicine is one of the first stumbling blocks encountered by the Westerner seeking to master its principles.

Here is the second obstacle for a Westerner: Chinese medicine is a philosophical medicine. In fact, the Chinese strove to integrate their medicine not in an anatomical or biological context but in accordance with their philosophy; this means that basic medical principles include discussions of the forces of nature, balance among the elements, treatises on heat and cold, etc. In addition, sacred aspects of numerology were also employed in the study of medicine.

The Chinese have always been and remain fascinated by figures. One need only mention the "hundred flowers," the "band of four," the "four modernizations," and so forth. To the Chinese mind, the harmony of the world is based upon the combination of numbers. Five, nine, and twelve each have a range of esoteric associations, for instance, as well as correspondences in all the other domains of life: astronomy, agriculture, daily tasks . . . and medicine.

Corresponding to the five fundamental elements and the five cardinal directions (North, East, South, West, and the Center) are the five flavors, the five odors, and the five primordial organs of the human body. Everything combines this way in a perfect harmony that the Chinese mind finds to be the summit of satisfaction.

But this veritable osmosis of medicine and philosophy, satisfying as it may be to the Chinese mind, is not readily acceptable to the Western mind. In fact, its application brings into play rules of thought and reasoning that are quite different from the analytical and logical form of reasoning to which we are accustomed.

The rules for using Chinese medicine appeal to notions that seem purely speculative to us: points and meridians, wonderful vessels, ancestral or perverse energies; these are all words that bring to mind the animal spirits and "malefic virtues" of our medieval doctors.

Then there is a third shoal for the Western mind to negotiate: Chinese medicine is an esoteric medicine. Point selections and treatment strategies are often based on abstract, esoteric principles like the name of a specific point, or astrological calculations.

So how could a style of medicine with these three distinguishing features (contradiction, philosophy, and esoteric nature) not be antithetical to the Western medical mind, which is so specifically keen on deductive reasoning and scientific knowledge? How did things develop to allow a medicine like this to get a strong foothold in our part of the world?

The answer is simple: it is effective. This medicine with all its original features has traveled through 1,500 years of history unchanged, and survived this way until around the 1960s. It was in this way that it was able to reach the West by several successive channels. When used following the Chinese rules, acupoint therapy attacks illnesses and can improve or cure pathological states with an ease that is often disconcerting. More impressive is the fact that this medical modality is performed almost without any pain, toxicity, or medication. It has therefore gained the adherence of many Western doctors. But criticisms and sarcastic jibes have not been lacking. Let me just say that twenty years ago you needed a thick skin and a lot of belief in yourself to admit to being an acupuncturist. Then, all of a sudden, everything changed. And this change came—as it should have—from China, its land of origin.

The reasons for this transformation are threefold: first there was the attitude the Chinese authorities began displaying toward their own native medicine; all at once, a lot of time and energy went into rehabilitating it. Next, the medicine was taught to a maximum number of practitioners—the "barefoot doctors" charged with the distribution of treatments to the smallest villages in a population of one billion human beings. The last thing was the interest in seeing this medicine progress into domains that the ancestors could not even imagine. A program of practical and scientific research was developed, which prompted Chinese medicine to evolve considerably in the last several decades.

Although science still does not understand how or why acupuncture works, substantial insights into some of its features have been gained. These insights have occurred in four broad areas:

1. Discovery of some of the scientific mechanisms in acupuncture's effects
2. Discovery of new acupuncture points
3. Greater "specialization" of each point
4. New methods of working on the points

While these "discoveries" are still quite piecemeal, they are nonetheless fascinating, and well worth exploring in some detail.

1. The Discovery of Some of the Scientific Mechanisms in Acupuncture's Effects

I have already examined the essential points of this progress extensively in two of my earlier books: *How to Give Yourself Relief From Pain by the Simple Pressure of a Finger* and *How to Safeguard Your Health and Beauty by the Simple Pressure of a Finger*. I will therefore confine myself to providing a summary here with particular emphasis on the most recent developments.

It is in the field of pain that the most important advances have been made. It has also been demonstrated that the stimulation of the points trigger reactions on two levels:

- One is the level of the spinal cord where the painful sensation is blocked by a veritable "gate" that prevents its passage toward the brain. It was first believed that this blockage was electrical in nature and occurred at a specific level of the spinal cord, but this is not at all the case. There are several intermediary stages that are involved, during which the nervous system releases a chemical substance known as "substance P," whose purpose is to reinforce the sensation of pain. The stimulation of acupressure points blocks this release of substance P and therefore reduces the size of the pain message.

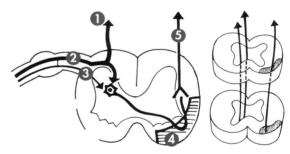

1. Fiber transmitting the pain sensation
2. Acupuncture inhibits the release of "substance P," blocks the sensation
3. Thicker "anti-pain" fiber
4. The "substance P" is blocked at several levels of the spinal cord
5. Ultimate sensation

The phenomenon of the gate

- Furthermore, a large number of neuropeptides are released in the brain by the nervous system; these mediators transmit the orders of one nerve cell to the next.

Among these are the endorphins—a kind of natural morphine that blocks the sensation of pain. It happens that acupuncture releases these endorphins, which explains part of its pain-mediating effect.

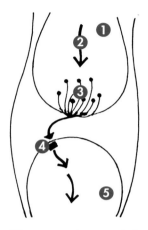

1. Upper neuron
2. Impulse arrival
3. Release of the neuropeptide
4. Neuropeptides collecting at a specialized site
5. Lower neuron

The transmission of the nerve impulse from one neuron to the other and the release of neuropeptides

In addition to this now well-established mechanism, there are no doubt many more that remain to be discovered. What we still don't understand about acupuncture includes:

- What passes through the mysterious meridians that crisscross our body?
- How do the acupuncture points communicate with brain receptors?
- Why do some points have an ipsilateral effect (on the same side of the body) and others a contralateral effect (on the opposite side of the body)?
- How does acupuncture act directly on the organs?

Acupuncture therefore opens an immense field of exploration across every aspect of our being. In this sense, you could say that it will be one of the royal ways of medical knowledge for the third millennium.

2. The Discovery of New Acupuncture Points

In classical Chinese medicine, there are as many acupuncture points as there are days in the year. But there are also hundreds of empirical and "extra" points that coexist with the classical meridian points. Some of these even have a very specific effect at specific times.

In addition to the classical points and empirical points, there are countless subsystems of acupuncture derived from different historical lineages—ear acupuncture, for instance, or Korean hand acupuncture.

Lastly, there are microsystems that envision the whole body holographically reflected in one of its parts—the ear, for instance, or the hand. Many of these microsystems use relatively "new" points that have been identified by experimentation, rather than historical precedent. The new points are often located on preferential treatment sites of the body: the sole of the foot, the palm of the hand, the scalp, the nose, and most particularly the ear.

3. The Greater "Specialization" of Each Point

This is one of the most important and the most interesting discoveries made by contemporary Chinese research.

The starting point for this research was

acupuncture-induced anesthesia. In the 1950s, Chinese doctors began to explore this new application of ancient healing methods. During the first operations performed in this way, dozens of needles were used, and a small army of assistants to keep the needles moving constantly during the operation. It is not hard to see how cumbersome this would be in an operating room and what kinds of difficulties it could cause.

Little by little, thanks to an enormous amount of experimentation (there have been more than three million operations performed under acupuncture anesthesia up to the present day in China), they were able to reduce the number of points to two, three, or a maximum of four during an operation. These were points that were found to have a demonstrable ongoing effect upon a given organ or region of the body. It was also found that electrical current directed to the needles would increase their effectiveness, and eliminate the need for continuous manual stimulation.

Many of the same points that have been demonstrated to work as anesthesia are recommended in this book for the treatment of diseases. They have, moreover, been divided and put into a hierarchy of principal points and secondary points. As I mentioned earlier, stimulation of the principal points is generally enough to obtain the desired effect; secondary points either reinforce or adjust this effect.

4. New Methods of Working on the Points

Traditionally, patients were treated on an ad hoc basis, in brief sessions at varying intervals. While attractive results could be obtained this way, many practitioners found they could achieve even better results with a series of treatments, each session lasting minutes at a time. These sessions could be conducted every day for a period of weeks and even months.

Methods of point stimulation were varied, but depended primarily on massage, acupuncture needles, and the application of heat in the form of burning incense—a technique known as *moxibustion.*

Moxibustion: an incense cone (mugwort, as a rule) on a protective layer (most often a slice of ginger).

As a further refinement, magnets or tiny seeds could be taped to the skin for more long-lasting stimulation. Nowadays, tiny intradermal needles can be inserted under the skin to remain there during the whole course of treatment. This is only one of the new ways of creating a semi-permanent stimulation; in fact, Chinese researchers have discovered multiple new ways of stimulating acupoints. For example, they now suggest the use of suction cups, little hammers equipped with many points, surgical incisions, or the placement of staples or threads that the surgeon can use to make sutures.

A variety of other methods have also been

tried, such as the application of magnetic discs on the points or injections of essential oils or medications at their location.

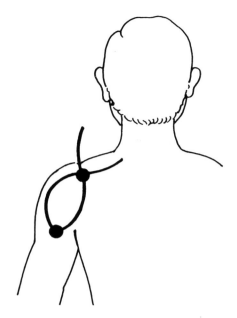

Placement of ligatures at several acupuncture points

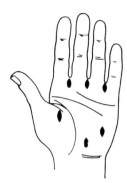

Several surgical incisions made at acupuncture points on the hands

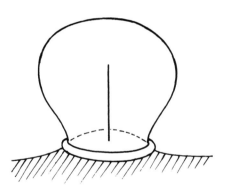

Placement of a suction cup over an acupuncture needle

The most prominent of these new methods is electrical stimulation, which is currently enjoying a considerable expansion. The administration of electric current can be done in two different ways:

• Small electrodes can be plugged into an electro-acupuncture unit. These electrodes can then be clipped to needles that have already been inserted into the skin. This is the practice used in surgical anesthesia. After the needles have been put in and connected to the electrodes, the current is turned on and its effect upon the patient lasts through the entire operation. This operation is painless and the patient remains conscious during it; he or she can even talk, drink, or eat during this time. This is a taxing and intensive method that should only be used by qualified medical professionals.

• Electrical current can also be applied directly to the skin. A number of small appliances have been invented for this purpose over the last several years. Until recently, these instruments were generally unreliable because they were either not sensitive enough or they were, to the contrary, overly responsive, wildly broadcasting their effects. But enormous progress has been made and the newer models of electric stimulators are quite accurate. The availability of reliable instruments means there is also now a treatment method available that is both simple and flexible. In addition, piezo-electric and laser stimulators are generally safe for lay-people to use, and are widely available.

In short, the power of acupuncture can now be partially harnessed by nonprofessionals using a variety of simple, safe, stimulation techniques. These methods require no medications but use only the natural healing reactions of the patient. Treatment is readily available to everyone as it presents no danger and is convenient to use. It can be combined with any other therapy or therapies and there are absolutely no contraindications.

This book is geared toward the at-home practice of acupressure stimulation, as this is undoubtedly one of the primary paths the practice of medicine will take in the future; it is a path that I believe will take a privileged place in the struggle against disease.

In fact, acupressure stimulation fulfills three conditions that, in my opinion, give it a notable advantage:

1. It prevents, totally or partially, the use of medication—especially the dangerous self-administration of chemical pharmaceuticals.
2. It permits the patient to take responsibility for health and healing into his or her own hands—literally—without discounting the role of medical doctors.
3. It represents the very spirit of preventive medicine, which can provide great benefit to millions of people. This is my personal motivation, and one of the reasons for writing this book is to offer this possibility to my readers.

While it is likely that acupuncture with needles done by a qualified professional will be more effective than at-home stimulation, there is still an enormous benefit to home treatments. They provide a first line of defense against disease, encouraging prevention and early treatment and thereby lessening the need for professional consultations.

NOTES FOR AT-HOME PRACTICE

As you begin to use the treatments described in this book, it will be helpful to bear a few things in mind.

The Power of Principal Points
As mentioned elsewhere in this introduction, the principal points suggested here are generally enough to treat a specific condition. If the patient does not respond sufficiently to the principal points, or if further specification would be helpful, then the secondary points are available.

Point Location Made Easy
I have described in simple terms the location of each acupoint, and have included detailed illustrations to help you find them. However,

a few of the points will be easier to find if you are able to first locate some basic body landmarks.

Specifically, several acupoints on the back are located in reference to the seventh cervical vertebra. This vertebra is most easily located by asking the patient to prop themselves up on their elbows and rotate their neck from side to side. This vertebra will be felt to rotate slightly. The first thoracic vertebra, which is the next vertebra down and the most prominent vertebra at the base of the neck, will not be felt to move during rotation. Count down one "bump" at a time from the seventh cervical vertebra to find the first thoracic vertebra, second, third, fourth, and so on.

Several other points are located in reference to the iliac crests. These are the prominent bones at the top of the hips. To find them, place your flattened hand in the depression at the side of the waist, with your pointer finger against the bottom of the rib cage and your little finger against the top of the iliac crest. This can be done with the patient lying on her front or her back. Then simply slide your hand across the torso keeping your little finger at the level of the top of the iliac crest. Locate your points on that line.

PART ONE

The Sense Organs

Conjunctivitis

CONJUNCTIVITIS IS AN inflammation of the outer membrane of the eyes, known as the conjunctiva. The principal sign of conjunctivitis is red eyes. But look out! Not all red eyes are conjunctivitis. Infinitely more serious eye diseases such as glaucoma, iritis (inflammation of the iris), and keratitis (inflammation of the cornea) can also make the eyes red. So if there is even the slightest doubt about the cause of this symptom, it is essential to consult an ophthalmologist.

When a person has conjunctivitis, the eyes will be runny, with a secretion that is more or less purulent and yellow or greenish in color. As a general rule, light does not overly irritate those stricken with conjunctivitis and the eye does not involuntarily shut when exposed to light; in other words there is little or no "photophobia." This is one way to eliminate the other more serious causes of red eyes. In some cases, small fluid-filled blisters may be noticeable on the conjunctiva. This is almost always indicative of an allergy.

CAUSES

There are three principal causes of conjunctivitis:

1. Infection by microbes. This was once almost the only cause of conjunctivitis. While it has not disappeared entirely, it is now much less common a factor than the other causes described below.
2. Allergy. This is now a frequent origin of this disease. Allergic conjunctivitis most often occurs in spring (though not always), and is sometimes accompanied by hay fever.
3. Viral infection. This is the most frequent cause of conjunctivitis today—herpes infections in particular. The virus that customarily creates a burning sensation or fever blister on the lips during a cold or

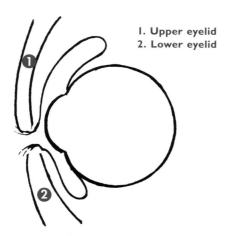

1. Upper eyelid
2. Lower eyelid

The conjunctiva covers the backs of the eyelids and the surface in front of the eye by creating two cul-de-sacs above and below.

other illness now strikes the conjunctiva with increasing frequency. It can cause a great deal of damage, especially as the treatment of it is quite difficult.

STANDARD TREATMENT

Treatment depends on which one of the three primary causes is responsible. Antibiotic eyedrops work extremely well in cases of infectious conjunctivitis, while cortisone eyedrops are effective in the cases with allergies. On the other hand, the treatment of viral conjunctivitis is extremely difficult, especially as the use of cortisone eyedrops—prescribed in error for this condition—can create a real disaster in the form of an ulcerated cornea.

ACUPOINT TREATMENT

While acupoint therapy is only useful as an accessory therapy in cases of infectious conjunctivitis, it can be quite helpful in treating viral and allergic cases. Here, the diligent and regular stimulation of the points brings about results that are often superior to other therapies and have none of the drawbacks.

TECHNIQUES TO USE

In the acute cases, short but intense stimulation for three to five minutes should suffice. In stubborn or recurring cases, however, what is called for are repeated stimulations two or three times a day, one to three minutes each time.

The Principal Points

The first is located on the inner corner of the eye by the tear duct; the second is on the back of the hand, in the angle formed by the bones that connect to the bones of the thumb and the index finger.

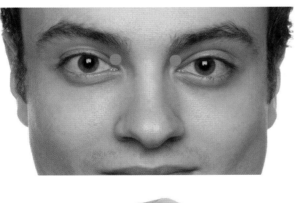
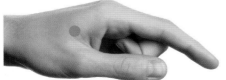
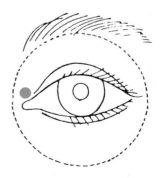
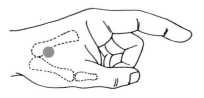

The Secondary Points

The first of the secondary points is located on the back edge of the skull, two finger-widths away from the ear, in a small indentation; the other can be found at the middle of the eyebrows.

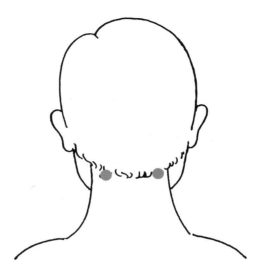

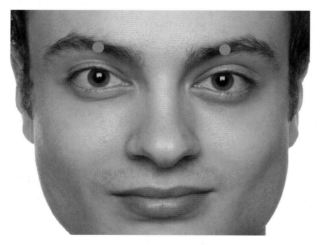

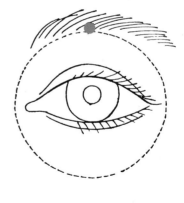

Glaucoma

GLAUCOMA IS CAUSED by a buildup of pressure inside the eye. In order to get a clear grasp of how it develops, we need to keep in mind the structure of the eye.

The eye contains two fluids. One—the vitreus humor—fills the space behind the lens and has the consistency of a gel. The other is the aqueous humor, which sits between the lens and the cornea. The aqueous humor has a fluid consistency similar to water, or to be more exact, a slightly salty serum. It is the elevation of the pressure on this fluid that creates glaucoma.

The aqueous humor is not a mass of stagnant fluid; it is constantly being secreted, and therefore expelled from the eyes—a little like a spring gives birth to a river. In some cases, the aqueous fluid becomes dammed up and the eyes are not able to filter or eliminate it: this is closed-angle glaucoma, which is responsible for the majority of acute glaucoma cases. In other cases, the source of the fluid releases too much and causes the tension to elevate gradually: this is open-angle glaucoma, responsible for the development of most cases of chronic glaucoma.

FORMS AND SYMPTOMS

Glaucoma comes in two forms: acute glaucoma and chronic glaucoma.

- *Acute glaucoma* comes on very dramatically. Suddenly the afflicted individual will feel a pain in his eye as if being stabbed with a knife. The eye then becomes red, taut, and hard as rock. This calls for emergency treatment: the sufferer should rush to the emergency room as quickly as possible to save his eyesight.
- *Chronic glaucoma* is much more insidious. The eye takes on a slightly pinkish hue and the eye feels not so much pain, but a constant irritation. Eyesight gets gradually blurrier either by continuous deterioration or in stages. The threat that chronic glaucoma poses to eyesight is less immediate than the acute form, but it is nevertheless quite real. Permanent damage can and should be avoided by getting medical attention as soon as possible.

Every case of glaucoma that is allowed to develop without receiving any treatment will inevitably lead to the loss of vision. It is therefore imperative that it be treated, and this treatment should be constant.

STANDARD TREATMENT

The crucial factor here is to lower the pressure in the eyes. In serious cases, this can be done through surgery. Generally, though, the use of medications that reduce the pressure in the eyes is sufficient, either administered by injection in emergency situations, or more commonly by eye drops.

In addition to the standard eye drops containing philocarpine, many people use beta-blockers. Whether these work better or not is unclear, but it is a rather demanding treatment that requires the patient to place eye drops, which are often an irritant, in her eyes every day.

ACUPOINT TREATMENT

We don't claim here that acupoint therapy can heal glaucoma, or recommend that it be used as a substitute for standard treatments. On the other hand, acupoint stimulation may allow a person to save money due to a reduced need for medication.

TECHNIQUES TO USE

For acute glaucoma, you need to get to the doctor without delay. On your way however, you can massage the eye points provided in this chapter. It's best to massage the points continuously without stopping. This can bring relief to the pain and sometimes even prevent impairment to the retina.

In cases of chronic glaucoma, a massage of the points should be repeated several times a day for about five minutes at a time, perhaps coordinated with the times you apply eye drops, for example.

The Principal Points

The first principal point is located in the inner corner of the eye next to the tear duct; the second is two finger-widths above the middle of the eyebrow on the forehead.

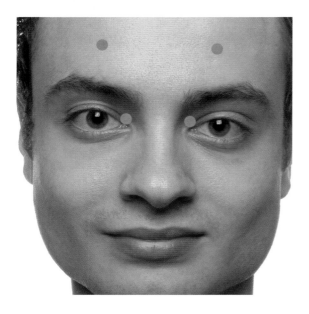

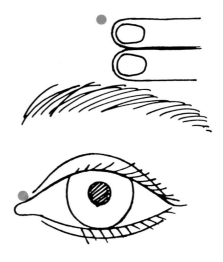

The Secondary Points

The first secondary point is located on the back edge of the skull, in a small indentation about three finger-widths from the back of the ear; the second is on the inside of the foot, on the calcaneum bone, a finger-width behind and below the tip of the ankle.

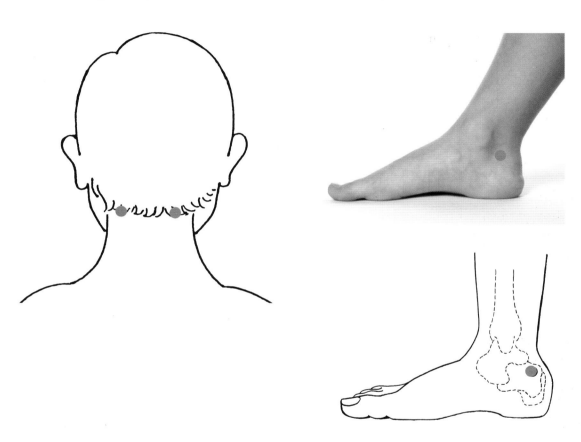

Myopia, Presbyopia, and Hyperopia

THESE THREE VISION problems—which are not diseases—are connected to the poor focalization of images on the retina.

Just what does this word, *focalization*—customarily used by photographers—mean? Focalization in regard to the eyes refers to the action of reproducing external images, at a reduced size, on the retina. (In fact, these images are also inverted—turned upside-down—though the brain will compensate for this and "flip" the image right side up.) What is most important are the clear contours that are achieved when the eye reproduces the object at the correct point on the retina.

Every schoolboy or schoolgirl has performed the experiment of concentrating the rays from the sun through a magnifying glass and catching the image on a sheet of paper. It is common knowledge that there is a precise distance, which varies depending on the curvature of the glass, at which the image of the sun is reduced to a dot—which sometimes sets the sheet of paper on fire. The same holds true for the normal eye, which is made up of transparent layers equivalent to our magnifying glass: the cornea, the aqueous humor, the vitreous humor, and the crystalline lens.

But if these layers—the glass itself—are either overly curved or too flat, it is easy to grasp how the perfect image would then form in front of or behind the retina. In these cases we are dealing with myopia (nearsightedness) or hyperopia (farsightedness). In all cases the image that is perceived will be out of focus, blurred.

Presbyopia, meanwhile, could be described as a kind of hyperopia linked to the aging process. Around the time most people turn fifty, the transparent layers of the eye—especially the cornea—become harder and lose some of their flexibility. This straightens the natural curvature of the eye, making it increasingly difficult for the eye to focus on close objects, which is the main symptom of presbyopia.

SYMPTOMS

The clearest sign of all of these deformities is vision trouble. The myopic sees things that are close quite well, and sees things that are far away quite poorly. The hyperopic sees what is far away quite well and has trouble seeing things that are close. This is also true for the person suffering from presbyopia; the first sign is usually the telltale fact that he or she has to hold the newspaper or book

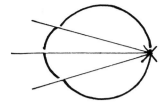 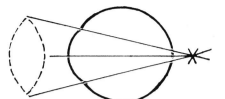 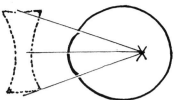

Normal eye:
the image is reproduced
correctly on the retina.

Hyperopic or presbyopic eye: the
image is made behind the retina
and requires a convex lens to be
corrected.

Myopic eye: The image is
made in front of the retina
and requires a biconcave lens
to be corrected.

they are reading farther and farther away in order to see it clearly.

CAUSES

In the great majority of cases, these problems of focalization are hereditary, and often present from birth. But the education system plays a huge role in revealing the existence of these eyesight problems by forcing children to constantly shift focus from the blackboard back to their notebooks. A child does not often realize he is not seeing properly, or else he cannot communicate it effectively. Many "lazy students" are primarily children who have trouble seeing.

Troubles related to focal points do not have a tendency to improve over time. On the contrary, they tend to worsen, and can even be the cause for serious accidents to one's sight. For example, strong myopia is often the origin of detached retinas, which can threaten a person's ability to see at all.

STANDARD TREATMENT

The standard remedies have a very long history: the wearing of corrective glasses with concave lenses for the myopic eye, and convex lenses for the individual afflicted with farsightedness or presbyopia, both of which artificially restore the focalization of the image. The eyeglasses that incorporate these solutions are a familiar feature of our everyday life.

In more recent times, the lens has been brought closer to the eye itself with the invention of contact lenses. In the beginning these were difficult to put in and were unpleasant to wear, but they have become more and more practical and easier to apply.

It is certain that the future of the standard treatment lies in the perfection of these "contacts," both in the material from which they are manufactured (plastic, silicon) and in the way they are cast so that they will be able to correct the slightest visual defect.

But we have now reached a point where the medical profession is attacking the very nature of the problem and audacious surgeons are "planing down" the very eye itself to correct these flaws in its curvature. These interventions—most popularly done with lasers—undoubtedly represent one of the paths to the future that may liberate the individual from subjugation to glasses, which have a tendency to get warm and mist over, to be irritating, to get lost, and so forth—in a word, they are merely prostheses.

ACUPOINT TREATMENT

Here is one group of problems where our stimulation points do not seem at first glance to have any role to play. And yet, the operations that I mentioned above clearly indicate that the disorder is physical and can be improved.

Where our efforts can bear fruit is by reducing eyesight problems, starting with children especially, and by delaying the onset of presbyopia to a riper old age.

TECHNIQUES TO USE

As these are not acute conditions, it is entirely suitable to stimulate the principal points for several minutes at a time, once in the morning and once in the evening—either by finger, needle, or electrical device. One sign of the effectiveness of these points is a numbing sensation in the eye. The achievement of this effect is a sign that the stimulation is working, and therefore helping to delay and reduce the deformity of the ocular curvature.

The Principal Points

The first point is located at the inside corner of the eyes, at the spot where tears begin to flow. Electrical acupuncture provided to this point offers extraordinary results, though it can also be stimulated manually.

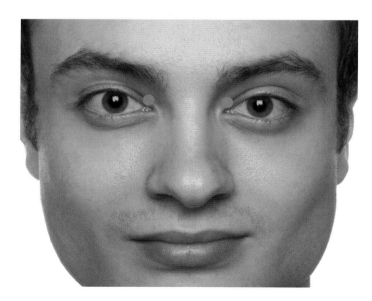

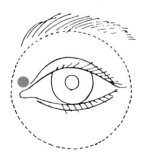

The second principal point is on the back
of the head, in a small hollow two finger-
widths from the side of the ear.

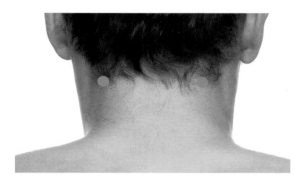
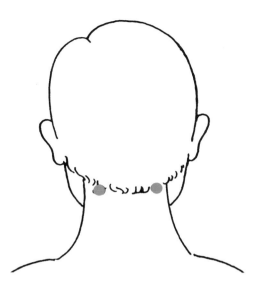

The Secondary Points

The first of these is located in the middle of
the eyebrow; the second is directly below this
point at the middle of the lower edge of the
orbit.

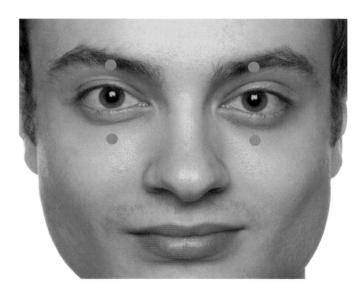
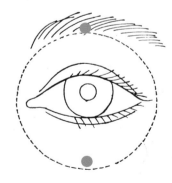

Retinal Disorders

THE RETINA APPEARS in the form of a film or a "skin" that lines the back of the eye. As the eye is essentially a ball, we can visualize that its back is a hemisphere whose concavity is facing forward. It is precisely this concavity that the retina carpets. In fact, this "film" is the flowering of the optic nerve.

The retina receives images from the outside and transmits them to the brain. To perform this function it has two categories of cells known as photoreceptors: cones and rods. Cones are responsible for the reception of colors while rods are responsible for receiving shapes.

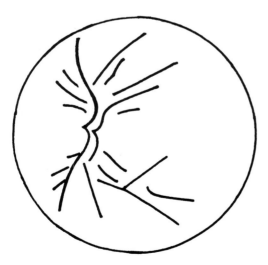

A view of the retina as it appears to the ophthalmologist, with the artery and vein of the retina.

If we add that this entire nerve complex receives its blood from one artery that accompanies the optic nerve, we can begin to grasp just how complex the visual system is. We should also note that because this artery comes from deep inside the head, observation of it is enough to give us a good general idea of the state of the arteries in the brain; it thereby offers us a very simple means of evaluating cerebral circulation.

FORMS AND SYMPTOMS

The retina can be affected in its anatomical entirety as well as in its nerve or vascular components.

In the first case, the most frequent disorder is a detached retina. This is actually a rip in the organ, though generally only a partial one. The only real symptom of this condition is the sudden appearance of brilliant sparks and flashes in your vision. It calls for quick intervention, because your eyesight can be permanently damaged. The most frequent cause—but not the only one—is strong myopia.

In other cases the retinal nerve itself is afflicted, in a condition known as retinitis. The disorder can cause things to look fuzzy and out of focus; objects may look as if they have been "erased" or distorted. The origin of retinitis is almost always a toxin, and among these toxins the most common culprits are alcohol and tobacco—or a combination of the two.

Finally, the arteries of the retina are also a common location of disease. The central artery or one of its branches can become clogged. This can be either temporary in the case of a spasm, or permanently in the event of a clot. While a temporary spasm may give rise to the black spots known as "floaters" in a patient's field of vision, a blood clot in the retinal artery can cause permanent partial or total blindness.

STANDARD TREATMENT

In the presence of so many different afflictions and causes, standard treatment of eye disease is necessarily quite varied. The normal treatment for a detached retina is almost always surgery, especially in serious cases. But considerable progress has been made using laser surgery for this condition. The laser ray essentially "glues" these small rips back together, and thereby arrests any further adverse developments.

Vascular disorders are also an emergency situation and require rapid dilation of the arteries to relieve the spasm or remove the clot. On the other hand, standard medicine is much less efficient at treating retinitis. Sometimes vitamins B_1, B_6, and B_{12} are prescribed in hope of restoring some vitality to the nerve.

ACUPOINT TREATMENT

Acupoint therapy has a fairly limited but important place in two extreme cases. The first is in response to a sudden onset of blindness where, while waiting to see the doctor, the vigorous stimulation of these points can save your vision. The other case would be retinitis, where in the absence of any valid treatment, the regular stimulation of the indicated points can have a noticeable effect.

TECHNIQUES TO USE

Doctors in China have no hesitation about treating acute cases by sticking long needles into the orbit of the eye socket. Of course this is not something that should be attempted at home or anywhere without the supervision of a trained professional! But vigorous stimulation of the point described below with your finger or an electrical device can also have potent results. If you are suffering from this kind of affliction, then you should massage this spot ceaselessly until the ophthalmologist can take over.

For a chronic disorder like retinitis, or as a complement to laser surgery treatment, repeated stimulation of these points for several minutes at a time, two or three times a day, can often help reduce lesions.

The Principal Points

The first point is located at the inside corner of the eyes, at the spot where tears begin to flow. Electrical acupuncture provided to this point offers extraordinary results, though it can be stimulated manually as well.

The second principal point is on the lower edge of the orbit, at a point one-third away from the outside and two-thirds away from the inside. This point, which is of recent discovery, is of considerable importance, and the Chinese have reported brilliant results from stimulation of it— even with people suffering from total blindness.

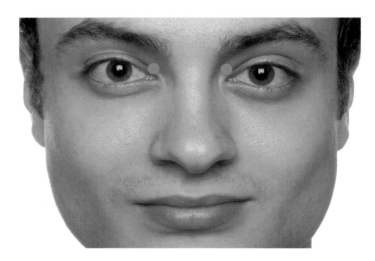

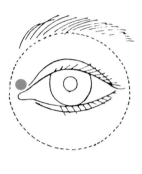

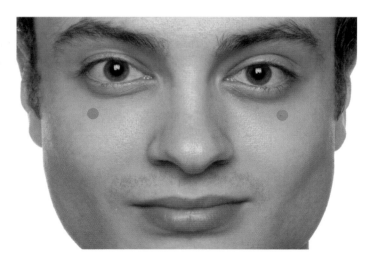

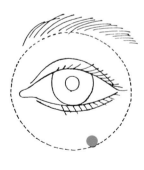

The Secondary Points

The first of these secondary points is on the back edge of the skull, in the hollow two finger-widths behind the top of the earlobe. The second point is located on the back of the hand inside the angle formed by the extensions of the index finger and the thumb.

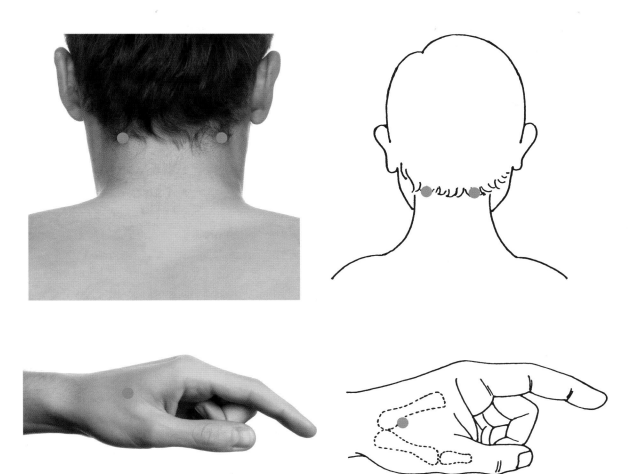

Strabismus

STRABISMUS IS A lack of binocular vision due to asymmetrical motion of the eyes. Whatever direction your eyes are looking in, they should be rigorously symmetrical. When this symmetry is not achieved, the resulting squint or cross-eyed appearance is known as strabismus. The only distinguishing feature in this condition is that the ocular globe can be pointing outward (external strabismus or wall-eyed) or inward (internal strabismus or cross-eyed).

To get a good grasp of the causes of the different forms of strabismus, you have to keep the functioning of the ocular globe in mind. This globe literally "floats" in a fluid environment composed of fat, located in the facial cavity that makes up the socket of the eye.

There are no less than six muscles involved in providing mobility to the eye, four of which enable it to move firmly in any one of four directions: up, down, inward, and outward. These are known as the rectus muscles. The last two muscles—oblique muscles—allow the eyeball to move when the head is moving. They act as pulleys, helping to keep the eyes stable as they change direction. Normally the movements of both eyes are strictly synchronized, with the "computer" that controls them located in the brain.

It is easy to understand how the movements of the eyes would diverge if for any reason one of the muscles should prove too weak to perform its duties. When this happens, the individual will begin to "squint" or look cross-eyed.

CAUSES

There are two major causes of strabismus. Among adults it is generally the byproduct of a cerebral disorder. This can occur following a viral attack or a small hemorrhage, at which point the afflicted individual suddenly begins seeing double.

In children, on the other hand, strabismus appears at a very early age—usually during the first months of life. It may be caused by a malformation in the muscles,

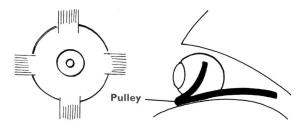

The four rectus muscles (left); an oblique muscle with its pulley (right).

which can be either too long or too short, or by a poor cerebral "mounting," in which parallelism has not been established. Whichever the cause, intervention is required as soon as possible. In contrast to the adult who is always extremely irritated by the double vision characteristic of strabismus, the child will quickly become accustomed to his handicap. He or she will put one eye to sleep in some way, and become used to looking at things only with the other eye. However, binocular vision is absolutely essential for precise determination of distances.

STANDARD TREATMENT

Even just a few years ago the only treatment prescribed for strabismus was generally surgery. The surgeon would simply alter the muscle that was too short or too long. But substantial development in medical therapies and physical therapy have considerably reduced the need for surgical intervention.

Adult double vision most often heals on its own, with or without the help of medications treating blood circulation. On the other hand, there are several effective vision therapies for childhood strabismus. These include eye exercises in which the good eye is covered by an opaque glass, so that the child must learn to use the other. With patience and tenacity, normal vision can be restored.

ACUPOINT TREATMENT

In adult strabismus or diplopia (double vision), acupoint therapy helps the vision return to normal. In childhood strabismus, the stimulation of points is a powerful aid in the re-education of the eyes, often shortening the course of therapy.

TECHNIQUES TO USE

There are two treatment points common to all cases of strabismus, and then two separate sets of points that are specific for inward strabismus or outward strabismus.

In cases of adult strabismus or diplopia, it's best to act quickly. Stimulate the points for several minutes at a time, every half hour until the vision returns to normal.

In childhood cases, stimulate the points in the mornings and evenings for two or three minutes at the end of any prescribed exercises.

The Principal Points

The first principal point is located on the back of the head, in a small hollow at the edge of the skull, two finger-widths away from the auricle of the ear.

The second point is located on the back of the hand in the angle formed where the thumb and index finger bones meet.

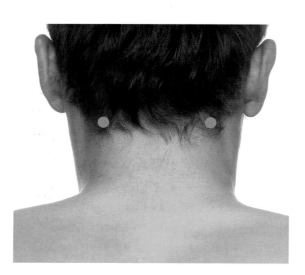
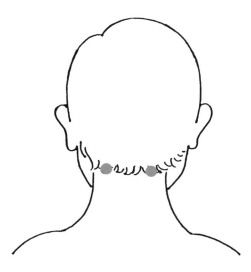

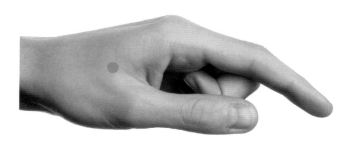

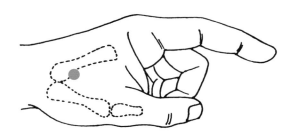

The Secondary Points

For inward strabismus, add the point located at the inner corner of the eye next to the tear duct and the point located in the middle of the eyebrow.

For outward strabismus add one point located at the outer edge of the eyebrow, halfway between the eyebrow and the hairline.

Add another point located on the inner edge of the orbit, at the junction located one-third of the distance from the outer edge and two-thirds of the distance from the inner edge.

The multiple number of these points suggests that electrical stimulation will be particularly effective.

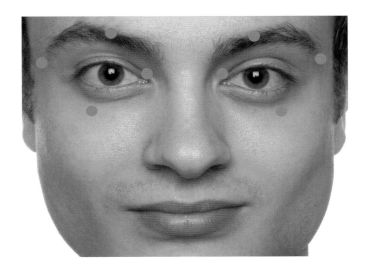

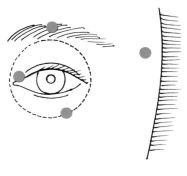

Deafness

BECAUSE SOUND, LIKE all sensations, is perceived by the brain, deafness can be caused by anything that interferes with the process of sound traveling from the outside world to those portions of the brain specifically designed to receive it. We should therefore take a look at just what this path consists of, and look at those obstacles that can occur along its course. When we talk, it is always in terms of one ear. However anatomists make a distinction between three sections of the ear, and the auditory nerve:

• The outer ear, which extends from the outer edge of the ear to the membrane of the tympanum or eardrum

• The middle ear or barrel of the ear (tympanic cavity), in which are found the little bones that transmit sounds

• The inner ear, which contains the centers that register sound and also the centers of balance

• Finally, the nerve that extends from the ear—the auditory nerve that conducts these sensations to the brain

Some obstacles to hearing occur in the outer ear, when the ear canal is blocked by a foreign object. This might be a small thing that a young child has inserted into his ear, for example, or even earwax, which in adults and children can harden and obstruct the ear canals. I have even seen a small spider and its web in this location!

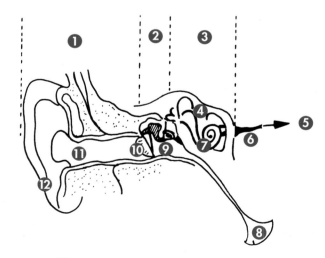

1. Outer ear
2. Middle ear
3. Inner ear
4. Semicircular canals
5. Toward the brain
6. Auditory nerve
7. Cochlea
8. Eustachian tube
9. Ossicles
10. Tympanum (eardrum)
11. Ear canal
12. Auricle

The ear

Two major problems can occur in the middle ear: otitis media (inflammation) and otospongiosis. Sometimes inflammation of the middle ear will cause an acute earache whose onset is dramatically accompanied by pain and fever. On the other hand, there are often small ear inflammations that develop without much fanfare. The most common sign of these is the secretion of a sticky viscous fluid from the ears. Serous earaches are a veritable "liquid" cork that deadens sound. If they develop unchecked, these kinds of ear inflammations will cause the eardrum to shrivel and eventually retract, which is a major cause of deafness.

Otospongiosis, on the other hand, is a malady that afflicts the tiny ossicles that transmit sound. Despite their minuscule size, these ossicles are connected to each other by actual joints. Sometimes one of these articulations will become blocked and two bones will knit together, preventing sounds from being transmitted in their full range and subtlety.

As different as these two disorders are from each other, the causes of hearing loss and deafness we have just discussed are both related to transmission; they involve a blockage affecting the transmission of sounds.

On the other hand, hearing loss that is caused by an attack upon the auditory nerve or the organs of the inner ear is referred to as hearing loss via perception: the illness affects the perception of sound. This kind of hearing loss can be the result of microbial infections, virus attacks, or small hemorrhages.

It can also be caused by a malformation or deterioration of the auditory nerve. This is often a consequence of growing old (and why the elderly often become "hard of hearing"). But there are hereditary forms that strike the very young. Finally, deafness can be a consequence of birth—the result of a malformation or infection suffered by the mother during her pregnancy.

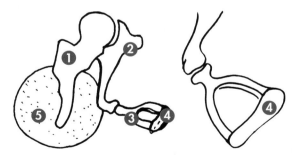

The Ossicles:
1. Hammer (malleus)
2. Anvil (incus)
3. Stirrup (stape)
4. Round window
5. Eardrum (tympanic membrane)

Detail of the anvil-stirrup (incus-stape) joint. Otospongiosis occurs when this articulation knits together. The operation to correct this condition consists of inserting a plastic ring between the two bones.

STANDARD TREATMENT

Earwax can be extracted by using a water jet (though never, never any metal object!), but the illnesses of the middle ear—inflammations, and shrinkage of the eardrum—are the specialty of the surgeon. In our lifetime we have witnessed the birth of a wonderful surgery that treats otospongiosis using a microscope.

Treatment for afflictions of the inner ear, on the other hand, are strictly of a medical nature. The subtle hearing loss connected to circulatory disorders represents a real emergency situation that calls for the rapid use of vessel dilators. But when the auditory nerve is damaged, there is nothing to do but use hearing aids. While these have become increasingly smaller and more effective, they can never truly replace the natural organ itself.

ACUPOINT TREATMENT

Here is an area where there was no expectation for results from acupoint therapy. However—and this is one of the major discoveries of contemporary acupuncture—it is surprisingly effective, not upon the superficial hearing loss caused by problems with transmission, but on the much more serious forms of hearing loss, those of perception.

A Chinese doctor named Tchao Pou Yi was able to successfully restore hearing to deaf-mute children simply by stimulating a specific point on a daily basis. It is time that we in the West really considered this miraculous point (as well as all the others).

TECHNIQUES TO USE

The deafness point is one that is treated in China with very deep stimulation using a long needle, to which an electrical current is often added. This is the treatment given to deaf-mutes. But we are now able to use electrical stimulation through the skin, which can be done without needles. As deafness is a chronic affliction, it is necessary to stimulate the appropriate points regularly—several times a day for several minutes at a time, in order to improve or stabilize the hearing.

The Principal Points

The first principal point—a point that is famous in China for its potent effects in the treatment of deaf-mutes—is located on the nape of the neck, two finger-widths below the edge of the skull on the median line.

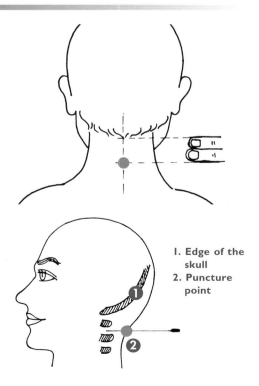

1. Edge of the skull
2. Puncture point

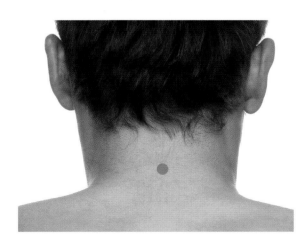

The second point is at the tip of the mastoid bone just behind the ear.

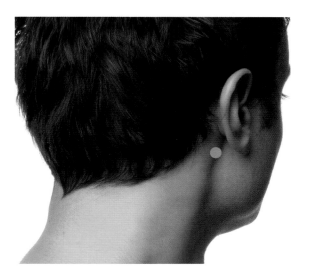

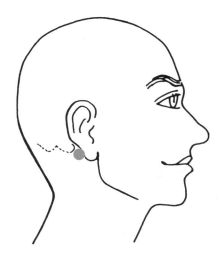

The Secondary Points

The first of these points is situated directly in front of the earlobe. The mouth has to be open in order to find it.

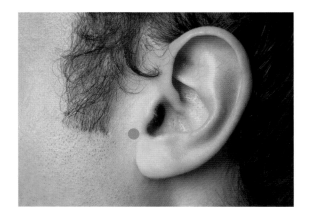

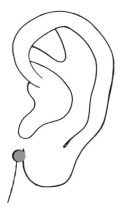

The Secondary Points (continued)

The second point is beneath the jaw, halfway between its two corners.

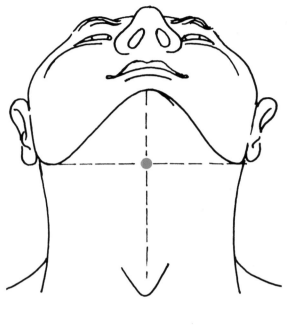

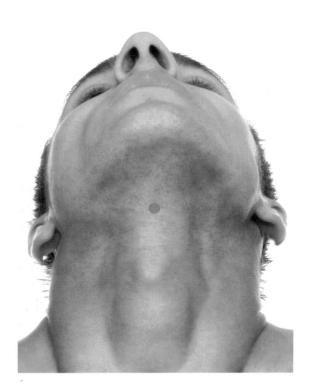

Tinnitus

TINNITUS DESCRIBES A chronic ringing in the ear, or any of those persistent noises perceived by the ears that have no objective reality. The person suffering from it may hear what sounds like metallic noises, explosions, or running water. But most often it is a ringing or whistling sound similar to the noise of a teapot boiling on the stove.

The noise can be continuous or intermittent, in the latter case often recurring at night. It can be accompanied by some loss of hearing and dizziness. In any event, for those who suffer from it, it can be an extreme annoyance and sometimes a social disability.

The ringing noises can appear suddenly, following directly after an attack of dizziness or exposure to a very loud noise. Sometimes, to the contrary, an abnormal noise gradually settles in and the patient cannot specify the time when his or her problem started.

CAUSES

The causes of tinnitus are unknown, and this annoying irritant still poses a difficult question for medicine. What *is* known is that tinnitus involves an irritation of the auditory nerve, but this irritation can occur among the nerve threads themselves or in the fluid areas of the ear: the labyrinth and semicircular canals.

Affliction by a virus is often cited as a cause, as is congestion of the nerve or a small clot in the arteries that feed it. Sometimes acute or repeated sonorous traumas can cause tinnitus, for example in workers whose jobs subject to them to loud noises—like jackhammer operators.

Unfortunately, once tinnitus has developed, it rarely subsides. Generally, the tinnitus sounds remain depressingly identical and last for an entire lifetime. Sometimes they get worse, and render life untenable for the individual suffering from them.

STANDARD TREATMENT

This is an easy treatment to sum up: there is no treatment. This is not for lack of trying. Sufferers have tried all kinds of products from blood dilators to products that are reputed to have an effect on the nerves. But to tell the truth, nothing yet has been found that works.

ACUPOINT TREATMENT

Acupoint therapy is all the more valuable as it often obtains very good results, though not in every case. When it's successful, such therapy can reduce or even eliminate the abnormal noises. It is therefore an excellent idea to stimulate the specific points systematically; even if they don't improve the condition, this therapy is harmless and offers no danger.

As this is a chronic affliction, it is helpful to repeat the stimulations for several minutes at a time, two or three times a day. I cannot emphasize too much how greatly electrical stimulation is indicated in this case.

TECHNIQUES TO USE

Electrical stimulation is particularly helpful for treating tinnitus. The device should be pressed steadily onto the skin.

The Principal Points

The first principal point is also a point used for treating deafness. It is located two finger-widths below the edge of the skull, on the midline. The second point is on the tip of the mandible behind the auricle of the ear.

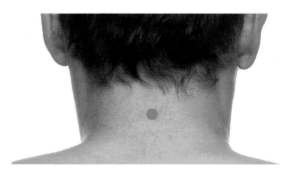

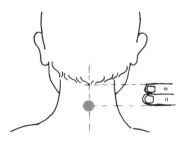

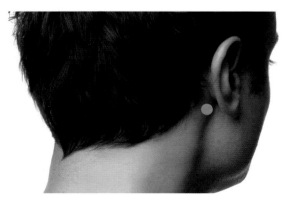

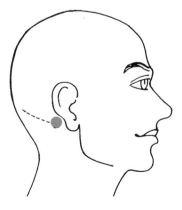

The Secondary Points

The first is on the top of the foot, between the big toe and its neighbor; the second is behind the inside of the ankle, just above the heel bone.

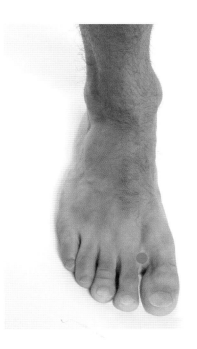

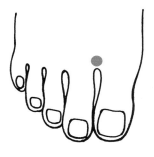

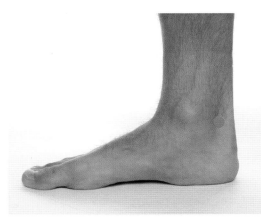

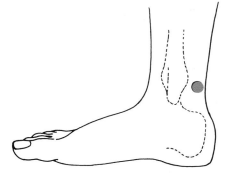

Vertigo

VERTIGO IS THE word most often used to describe dizziness. However, true vertigo is characterized by a sensation of spinning; it can feel like you are spinning around in the center of unmoving objects, or like you are seeing these unmoving objects revolving around you. Temporary "dizzy spells," on the other hand, may cause a person to feel unbalanced, and can be triggered by standing up too quickly or suddenly turning one's head.

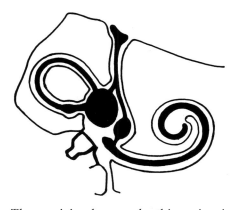

The semicircular canals: this region is called the cochlea, from the Greek word kokhlias, *which means "snail"—a good metaphor for this tube that is coiled like the spiral shell of a snail.*

CAUSES

There are two major causes for both true vertigo and simple dizzy spells: the ear and the spinal column.

The auricular kind of vertigo that accompanies Ménière's disease or head trauma is a dramatic form of dizziness that manifests with brutal rapidity and can be accompanied by tinnitus and hearing loss. The head keeps spinning no matter what position the patient adopts, even if he or she remains completely motionless. These heavy attacks of vertigo may also include vomiting and intolerable nausea. In such cases, the origin of the problem lies with an imbalance in the pressure of the fluid in the ear.

The inner ear contains the labyrinth with its semicircular canals—organs that are necessary for both hearing and balance.

It so happens that these tubes or canals contain fluid, the endolymph in the cochlear duct, which is separated from the surrounding bone by another fluid known as perilymph.

It is these semicircular canals—located at three different directions in space—which provide a sense of balance. Whenever there is excess fluid or a sudden drop in the pressure of the internal and external fluids, this sense is entirely disrupted, hence the attacks of dizziness.

Conversely, vertigo caused by the spinal

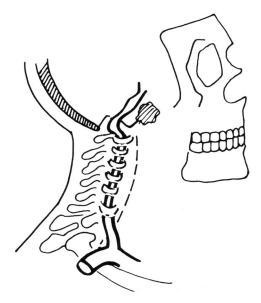

Vertebral artery: it is easy to see how the artery can get "pinched" inside the narrow spinal column.

column—also known as cervical vertigo—has a much less direct cause. It hinges on the vertebral artery, which passes through the seven vertebrae of the cervical spine. This artery just happens to feed the cerebellum, the part of the brain that is important for maintaining the body's sense of equilibrium.

If this artery should happen to get pinched inside the spinal column containing it, the cerebellum will experience a momentary interruption in its blood supply, and the impression of losing one's balance will follow. This is also sometimes described as vertigo from "shampooing," because it is easily produced when a hairdresser abruptly pushes one's head forward after washing the hair. This happens all the more readily when the spinal column is already abnor-mal with displaced vertebrae or deformities caused by degenerative arthritis.

Finally, vertigo or vertigo-like spells can also occur when blood pressure is abnormally low or in cases of serious anemia.

STANDARD TREATMENT

There are very few treatments for auricular vertigo, or for Ménière's disease in particular. Vascular dilators have been tried with very uneven results.

For cervical vertigo, a chiropractic adjustment by a highly skilled professional can improve the situation considerably.

ACUPOINT TREATMENT

Acupoint therapies also provide very uneven results, but because of their essentially innocuous nature, there is no reason not to try them, alone or in combination with other therapies.

TECHNIQUES TO USE

For Ménière's disease, the best procedure is to stimulate the principal points for a long time—from ten to thirty minutes several times a day.

On the other hand, a more modest stimulation of two or three minutes, two or three times a day, is sufficient for the vertigo or dizzy spells that are caused by the vertebral artery or by tension.

The Principal Points

The first principal point is located on the back of the hand in the angle formed by the two bones that go on to form the fourth and fifth fingers.

The second point is on the skull, five finger-widths above the top edge of the ear.

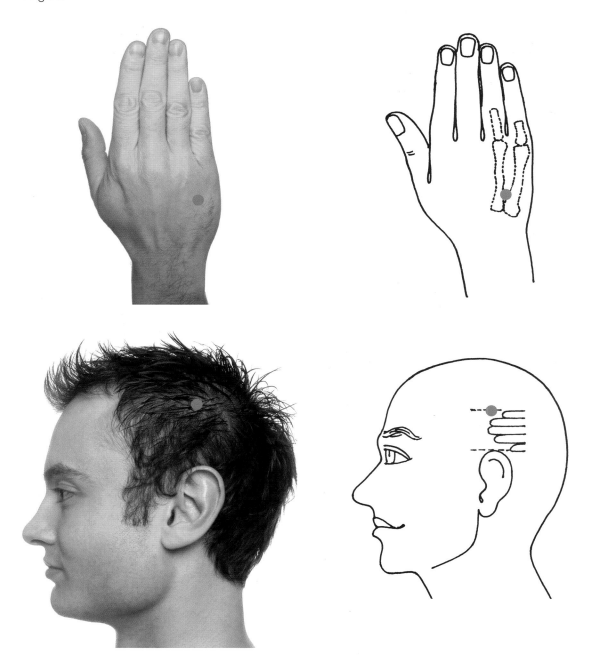

The Secondary Points

The first of these points is found on the back edge of the skull, in the small hollow two finger-widths from the back of the ear; the second is just in front of the ear, directly below the small protruding area called the tragus that comes to an end just in front of the ear canal.

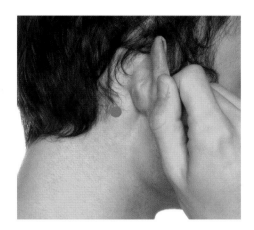

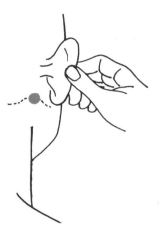

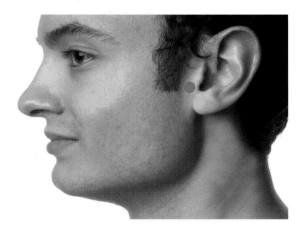

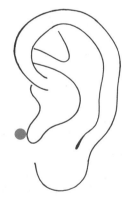

Head Colds and Rhinitis

WHAT COULD BE more banal than the illness that affects the most noble organ of the body: the head? The medical terms for head colds describe them more precisely as *coryza* or acute rhinitis, both of which pertain to inflammation of the mucous membranes inside the nose.

SYMPTOMS AND FORMS

Who is not familiar with the symptoms of a cold? A sudden onset announced by a burning sensation in the nose and throat, constant sneezing, nasal blockage followed by a stream of fluid that starts colorless but becomes green or yellow as it becomes more purulent. In addition, colds affect the neighboring organs. Often the eyes run, ears clog, and sometimes the cold goes down into the chest, which is to say it triggers an attack of bronchitis. But under normal circumstances, everything goes back to normal working order after eight to ten days.

What I described above, however, is the standard form, one that is generally benign. In a certain number of cases, things do not turn out to be so simple.

First, for nursing infants and very young children—whose lack of natural defenses, narrowness of nasal passages, and lying-down position causes a flow of pus into the bronchial tubes, the digestive tract, and the ears especially—colds are a purveyor of countless childhood infections, particularly ear infections. (I have personally known a young child who had to have his eardrums opened thirty-two times in one winter.)

Next, colds among school-age children amount to a veritable disability. Because they constantly come down with colds their overall state of health can be adversely affected; this can pose threats to their ongoing development, not to mention their ability to get a sound and well-rounded education.

Finally, rhinitis or nasal inflammation can become a chronic condition for some adults. Going from one cold to the next, these patients have chronic "sniffles"; their nasal passageways are always clogged and they always need to blow their noses. This then becomes an illness that affects one's entire life, by altering the sense of smell, causing constant headaches, and posing a permanent threat to the respiratory system, particularly the sinuses.

Did you know that acute or chronic colds may be the most expensive drain on the medical system and society as a whole, just by the work absences they cause?

CAUSES

Colds can be caused by bacterial or viral infections, both of which are legion in number. In addition, a bacterial infection can arise secondarily to a viral infection, infecting the nose again and causing more suppuration of its fluids.

Many conditions of our modern world encourage these infections and contagions: a moist climate, pollution, tobacco smoke, and crowding are the most frequent culprits. (Contagious diseases spread quite efficiently in places like day care centers, schools, and offices.)

But we need to add another cause to these: allergies—the inherited or acquired sensitivity to a number of things including dust, germs, and chemical products. Among these latter we have to highlight the danger posed by medicinal products in particular, especially nasal drops that are used far too often; it has reached a point that constitutes abuse.

The co-occurrence of infection with allergies can cause a vicious circle: infection-allergy-infection. The patient becomes the victim of a perpetual cold, and his permanently inflamed mucous membranes thicken as a result, thus further obstructing the nasal passages and respiratory tract.

STANDARD TREATMENT

The common head cold is the greatest shame and failure of contemporary medicine. Mankind knows how to fly to the moon but we still do not know how to cure a cold!

We are not even sure how to treat it. When you are following your grandmother's advice (protect yourself against cold temperatures, rinse the nose with salty water) you are at least not causing any great harm. But this is not true about vasoconstricting nasal drops; and it is certainly not true about using antibiotics. Who has not known a child who takes antibiotics every day from October to May, to the great distress of his or her digestive tract, growth, and teeth?

ACUPOINT TREATMENT

For the reasons noted above, the existence of a natural therapy that is effective but poses no other health risks is extremely helpful. Used at the very onset of a cold, stimulation of the points I've provided stops it "cold." Used after a cold has become established, they will still relieve its discomforts and will, to a large extent, arrest its development. For this reason, I recommend that our method be the one you try first, either by itself or in combination with other natural methods.

TECHNIQUES TO USE

When the first sensations of an incoming cold make themselves felt, intense stimulation for five or six minutes of the first three principal points should be enough to quell them.

Once a cold has established itself, or in the case of chronic nasal inflammation, it is necessary to repeat this stimulation in the morning and the evening for two to three minutes each time, in order to obtain relief.

The Principal Points

The first principal point is situated in the middle of the forehead just above the hairline. (If you place the base of your index finger at the bridge of your nose, your fingertip should reach this point located in a small hollow on the brow.)

The second principal point is located on either side of the nose, in the small hollow at the outside edge of each nostril.

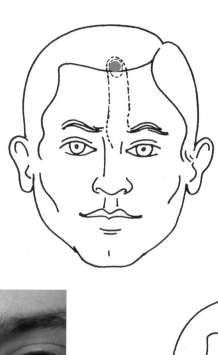

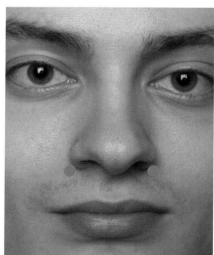

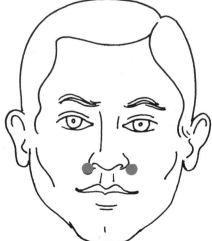

The Secondary Points

The first of these points is located in the nape of the neck over the spinal column, just beneath the bulge of the first thoracic vertebra, which can be found by running your finger down the spinal column starting from the nape of the neck.

The second point is above the bridge of the nose, just beneath the bony ridge that is located there.

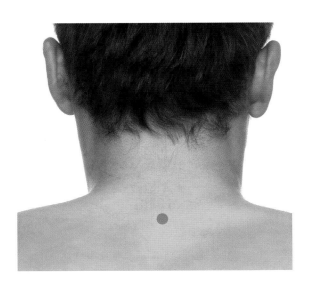

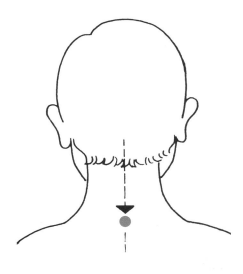

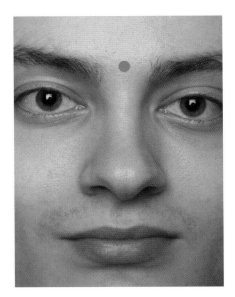

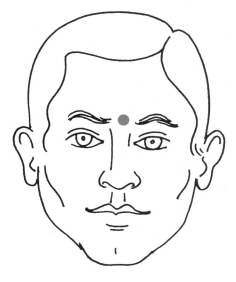

Acute and Chronic Sinusitis

SINUSITIS IS THE clinical term for an inflammation of the facial sinuses. This inflammation can be caused by irritations or allergens, or by infection. Like other infections, sinus infections can either be abrupt and acute, or chronic and long-lasting.

The sinuses are hollow spaces enclosed within the thickness of certain facial bones; they are connected with the nasal cavities. It has been said that their chief purpose is to lessen the weight of the facial bones, though that question is still under debate. In any case, they have no role in respiration although they are traversed by air.

There are three groups of sinuses: the frontal sinuses, the ethmoidal sinuses, and the maxillary sinuses. The first are located in the forehead beneath the eyebrows, at their inner edge. The ethmoidal sinuses or cells are located within the depths of the face and play a role of particular importance in children. The maxillary sinuses are in the cheeks.

SYMPTOMS

The signs or symptoms of sinusitis will vary depending on its location. Acute maxillary sinusitis is often a complication of a cold that appears around the third or fourth day of its development. The major symptom is the abrupt appearance of a sharp, throbbing pain located in the cheek directly below the eye. If it goes untreated it will persist with periods of relief interrupted by pain.

With or without treatment, maxillary sinusitis can be healed, but it quite often becomes chronic. In this event the pain disappears but a purulent and endless nasal drip remains.

Attacks of frontal sinusitis are even more painful, if that is possible, with sensations of stabbing pain radiating around the inner corner of the eye. This condition can also become chronic.

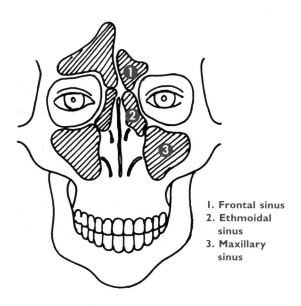

1. Frontal sinus
2. Ethmoidal sinus
3. Maxillary sinus

The sinuses

Finally, ethmoidal sinusitis is an affliction that especially targets infants and young children. The signs of its presence appear in the upper corner of the eye and around the upper eyelid, which abruptly becomes quite swollen. There are even sometimes cases when the eye is pushed forward, and can appear to be thrust out of its orbit.

CAUSES

Sinus infections are most commonly the result of a cold that blocks the sinuses with mucus. However, they can also be caused by allergies or fungi, or by irritation from pollutants such as cigarette smoke or smog. What explains the violent symptoms of sinusitis is the fact that the orifices that connect the sinuses with the nasal cavities are extremely narrow. They can become clogged almost immediately and the pressure this puts on the pus in the sinuses can trigger outbursts of pain.

In the chronic forms of sinusitis, a lingering infection and often an allergy can be the cause for relapses. There is also the possibility that a neighboring infection, particularly a dental infection, may be at fault.

STANDARD TREATMENT

The essential thing is to restore the permeability of the sinus canals. This can be achieved with vasoconstricting nose drops, which cause the sinus passages to dilate and thereby relieve the pressure. But these drops should not be overused because they will eventually become an irritant to the mucous membranes. Sometimes a patient will have to resort to local treatments of the kind only an ear and nose specialist can provide. Antibiotics are often combined with the treatment. If the discharge cannot be eliminated from the body through its natural channels, it is sometimes necessary to drain the pus surgically, through a puncture made in the skin and the bone.

ACUPOINT TREATMENT

Acupoint therapy is quite effective because it specifically addresses the essential cause of the disease—the obstruction of the sinus canals—and makes it possible for the sinuses to drain. It is always worth taking the effort to apply this therapy, and you will often have the satisfaction of seeing the mucus start flowing out of the nostrils during the very first time you apply stimulation.

TECHNIQUES TO USE

For acute sinusitis, the points need to be massaged quite energetically for a long time in order to obtain relief and cause the pus to be discharged. Massage the points deeply for ten to fifteen minutes, or until they begin to feel better.

For chronic sinusitis, it is enough to apply repeated stimulation for two to three minutes, in the morning and in the evening.

The Principal Points

The two principal points are the same ones that are used to treat colds (see page 44). The first point is on the forehead over the median line. Place the bottom of your index finger at the top of the nose and bend your finger in until it finds a small hollow in the bone. The second point is located at the outside edge of both nostrils.

The Secondary Points

The secondary points vary depending on which sinus is affected. For the *maxillary sinus*, the point is beneath the eye, right below the center of the orbit; for the *frontal sinus*, the point is in a small cavity at the inner end of the eyebrow.

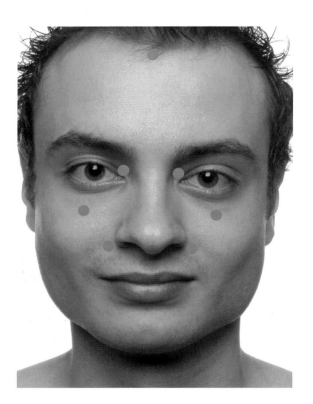

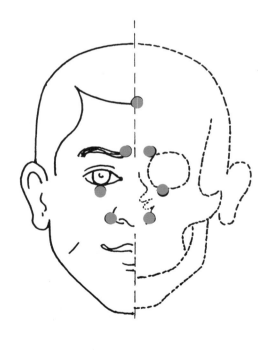

Flu and Nasal Congestion

IN THE STRICT sense of the term, the various kinds of flu are due to the influenza virus. But in common speech, the word *flu* often designates any infection of the throat and nose, even though it may actually have been caused by a different virus. Here we shall use the name *flu* to describe the constellation of symptoms, knowing that it is often quite difficult to pinpoint the virus that is responsible. Furthermore the therapies for these conditions, both the standard treatment and our methods, are the same regardless of the original cause.

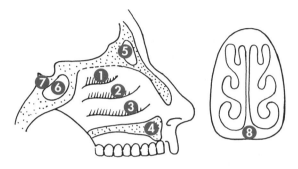

1. Upper turbinate
2. Middle turbinate
3. Lower turbinate
4. Hard and soft palate
5. Frontal sinus
6. Sphenoidal sinus
7. Turcic saddle
8. Nasal partition

At left, nasal cavity (cross section); at right, turbinates (vertical view)

SYMPTOMS

The symptoms of flu are well known:

- Sudden outbreak of a fever that can rise as high as 102° to 104° Fahrenheit
- A head cold, sore throat, and coughing
- General feeling of malaise, aching sensations in the limbs, headaches
- Swollen lymph nodes
- Often accompanied by digestive distress, diarrhea, vomiting, and so forth

While there is little value from the Western perspective in focusing on this or that aspect of the flu, it is useful to know that the Chinese medical mind sees the existence of two forms of flu:

- the *cold form* or the invasion form, with shivering, headaches, clogged nose, and scratchy sore throat;
- the *warm form* with flushed face, sweating, high fever, body aches, and coughing.

CAUSES

Flu is always caused by a viral infection. The course of an infection is generally benign: after a week or so the symptoms start diminishing, the fever breaks, and the patient recovers. But among individuals who are worn out, already ill, or elderly, the evolution of this disease can be quite a different story. Microbes can invade the body that the virus has already weakened, leading to the appearance of serious respiratory problems capable of killing the patient. Even today in our part of the world, the flu is still one of the biggest causes of death.

STANDARD TREATMENT

Just as with other viral diseases, there are no truly effective treatments from the standard allopathic medical practice. Bed rest, hot drinks, and fever-reducers are all simple palliatives. Vitamin supplements, which were strongly advocated for a while, have not been proven to be effective.

ACUPOINT TREATMENT

Acupoint therapy applied in the initial stages of flu can stop it from developing. However, it is necessary to catch it very early, and to clearly keep in mind the distinctions between the two forms described above.

TECHNIQUES TO USE

In the *cold* or invasion form of the flu, stimulate the points as soon as possible, once every hour, or use energy stimulation such as an electrical stimulation. In the already calmed stage or the *warm form,* stimulate the points two to three times a day.

A stimulation that has been performed in time (during the first half-day) can stop the development of the flu in its tracks.

The Points: Cold Form

In the cold form or invasion stage, there are three very important points. The first is the point between the tips of the shoulder blades, beneath the bony protuberance of the first thoracic vertebra.

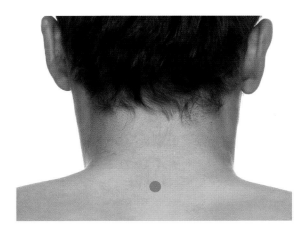

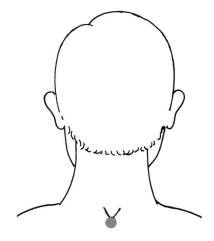

The second point is in the middle of the slope of the shoulders; the third, on the back of the wrist between the two bones of the forearm.

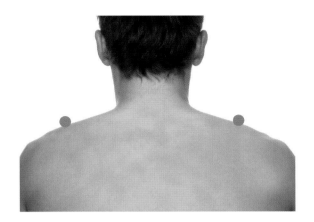
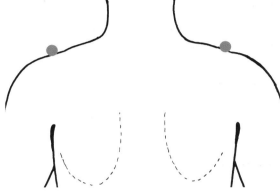
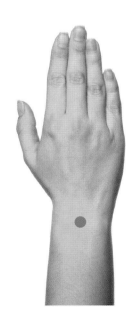
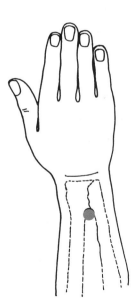

The Points: Warm Form

For the warm form there are also three sets of points. The first are on the nape of the neck behind the ears, in the first indentation the finger will find beneath the edge of the skull.

The second point is found at the junction of the nose and the forehead; the third set of points is located at the lower outside edges of the nostrils.

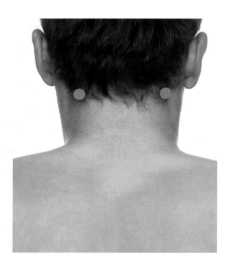

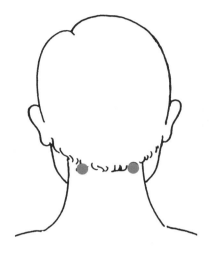

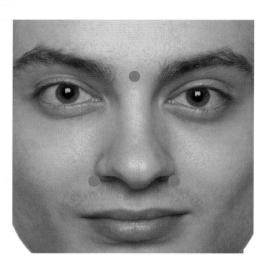

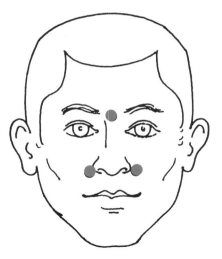

Gingivitis and Cold Sores

THERE ARE A good many diseases that can affect the tongue and mouth. I do not intend to review them all here, and will simply examine the most common ones, including gum disease or *gingivitis,* and cold sores that can affect the gums, the tongue, and the interior of the mouth.

SYMPTOMS AND CAUSES

The presence of gingivitis—an infection or inflammation of the gums—is generally betrayed by a painful swelling of the gums which become spongy, often bleed, and sometimes ooze pus. Infections are the most frequent cause of gingivitis. As a general rule, such infections usually begin in a neighboring area like the teeth or throat.

Infections and inflammations of the tongue are called *glossitis.* The tongue of someone with glossitis will typically appear smooth and glossy, as if its normal surface contours have been scraped away, particularly the papilla. Painful swelling or cracks on the tongue are signs of this ailment, which is often due to an organic or metabolic disorder connected to vitamin deficiency (particularly vitamins B_3 and B_{12}). But attacks by yeasts or molds are also a frequent cause. Particularly implicated is *Candida albicans*—the yeast that causes thrush in nursing infants, and is now increasingly afflicting adults, especially following antibiotic treatments.

Cold sores are another common affliction of the mouth and tongue; they are small ulcerations that can occur singly or in multiples. They cause a painful burning sensation and sometimes develop in successive eruptions that can be extremely irritating.

The cause of cold sores remains a mystery and all that is known for certain is that they are in no way related to the foot and mouth disease that affects animals. Whatever the cause may be, any mouth ulcer that does not heal should not be ignored, especially if the sufferer is a smoker. A doctor should be consulted.

STANDARD TREATMENT

The treatments for these kind of ailments are as varied as their origins. The most often used products are antibiotics and vitamins, depending on the circumstances. Lesions require diligent study and treatment from the start.

As for cold sores, we are forced to acknowledge that there are no currently valid treatments for combating them, other than various over-the-counter remedies.

ACUPOINT TREATMENT

With cold sores, acupoint therapy can have stunning results, ranging from rapid improvement to a complete cure. When it comes to gingivitis, the treatments might be best when combined with other therapies.

TECHNIQUES TO USE

When treating cold sores, the massage of the first point indicated should be deep and strong—with an electronic device or a fingertip. A session of electrical acupuncture can even block a cold sore eruption.

To treat chronic gingivitis, or to prevent future eruptions of cold sores, the sessions need to be repeated in the morning and in the evening, for several minutes each time.

The Principal Points

The first principal point is located beneath the chin, halfway between the two corners of the jaw. The second is on the back of the hand, inside the corner formed by the bones that lead to the thumb and index finger.

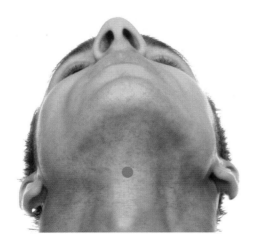

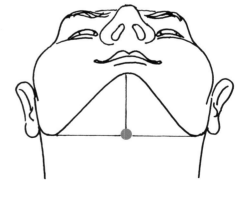

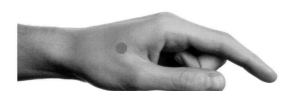

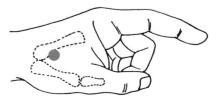

The Secondary Points

The first of the secondary points is one finger-width away from the corner of the jaw; the second is found at the end of the second toe on the side of the nail facing the outer edge of the foot.

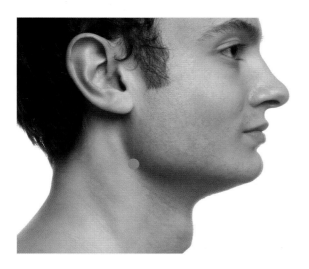

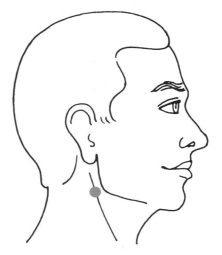

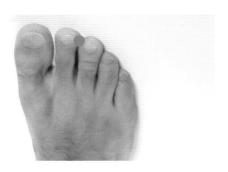

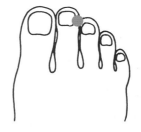

Toothache

DISEASES AND DISORDERS of the teeth have an entire branch of medicine of their own, and are too numerous and complex to be covered in great detail here. This is especially true because it is not only ailments of the teeth that concern us, but also the conditions that may affect the arrangement of our teeth in the jaw.

The teeth sit inside small hollow sockets in the bone called alveoli. A complicated system of "moorings" connects each tooth to its socket and is at risk of loosening, becoming infected, or disintegrating with age. This "arthritis," properly called *parodontosis,* has yet to find any totally satisfactory form of treatment.

SYMPTOMS

The number one sign of a tooth ailment is a toothache. This is a pain of the nerves and can be quite acute—a fierce stabbing pain. However, a mild to moderate case of parodontosis often has very little pain associated with it; nonetheless the teeth "move" and eventually fall out.

STANDARD TREATMENT

We shall not look at the standard treatments here in detail as all forms of dental care are highly specialized.

ACUPOINT TREATMENT

Acupoint therapy can be helpful both in the case of toothache and for parodontosis.

TECHNIQUES TO USE

These points should be stimulated strongly for the treatment of pain, until the symptoms recede. For chronic tooth afflictions, these points will require several minutes of massage, in the morning and the evening.

It is worth noting that these are also the points that dentists and acupuncturists specializing in stomotology (there are more and more of them) use to perform their dental treatments without the use of chemical anesthesia.

The Principal Points

There are two principal points. The first is located on the back of the index finger just outside the corner of the nail, on the edge facing the thumb. The second is on the outer end of the fold created when bending the elbow.

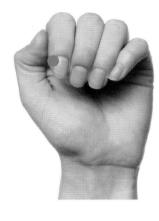

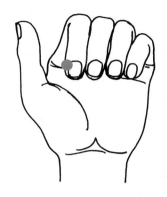

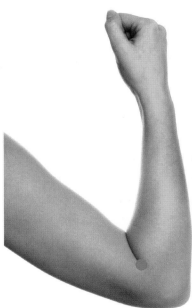

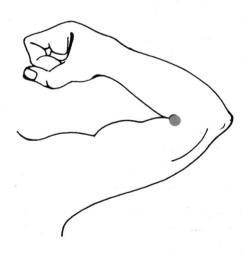

The Secondary Points

There are a number of secondary points that vary depending on which tooth is being treated. For the upper teeth: in all cases use the point found on the back of the hand in the angle formed by the two bones going into the thumb and the index finger.

There are two secondary points for the teeth in the lower jaw: one is located beneath the chin, midway between the two corners of the maxillary bone; the other point is situated on the jaw, about a finger-width above and in front of the corner, on the spot where the muscle juts out when you clench your teeth.

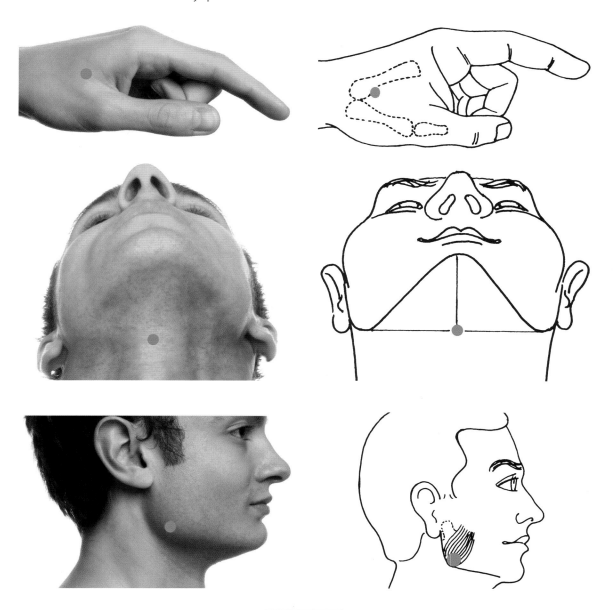

For molars, premolars, and the canine teeth, use the point located just beneath the cheekbone. For the incisors, use the point located at the middle of the upper lip beneath the nose.

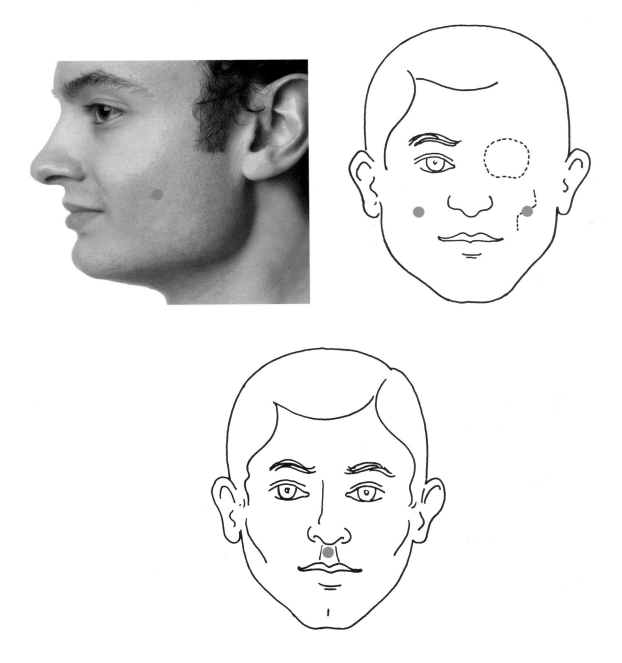

Sore Throat and Tonsillitis

ALL INFECTIONS OR inflammations of the throat are commonly referred to as a "sore throat." But the "throat" is not an anatomical term; it covers a whole series of territories including the soft palate, the pharynx, and the tonsils. So a sore throat could describe an inflammation in all or just a part of these territories.

Of all these structures, the tonsils are the most important. There is a great deal of confusion surrounding the role of these organs, which it is necessary to dispel. First, the tonsils that can be seen when you open your mouth are, in truth, just part of a larger circle that continues upward toward the nose and descends behind the tongue.

What is the value of this circle? It is quite simply a defense ring—a veritable fortress that has been erected at the entrance to the body, at the crossroads formed by the intersection of the respiratory and digestive tracts. This explains why the tonsils need to be saved whenever possible.

Large tonsils are not—especially in children—always abnormal; quite the contrary. This is where the child is going to construct a means of defense against infection. It is something we should really not mess with.

SIGNS AND SYMPTOMS

The most obvious sign is of course the kind of burning pain that is felt in the throat, a sharp or shooting pain that is aggravated by swallowing and can often make eating a hardship. It is often accompanied by a sense of general malaise and a low or moderate fever.

To an observer, the back of the throat will appear red and swollen. There may be small white spots on the tonsils, and sometimes even veritable membranes. Sometimes small bubble-like blisters like those of a nettle rash can be seen, which are the sign of a sore throat caused by a virus.

CAUSES

Germs in the mouth cause almost all sore throats. At one time, sore throats accompanied by a diaphanous membrane were one of the symptoms of diphtheria, which has almost vanished today. Nowadays, Vincent's Angina

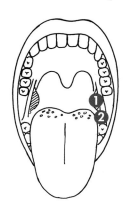

Tonsil (1) and tonsilar pillar (2)

is almost the only disease responsible for this symptom. As we saw above, the sore throats with blistering that can invade the bronchial tubes and esophagus are viral in origin. Most importantly, almost any sore throat can reveal the onset of more serious diseases like meningitis, rheumatism, heart diseases, and so on. Therefore it is a good practice to keep an eye out for the bacteria responsible for these ailments: streptococcus.

STANDARD TREATMENT

The standard treatment for sore throats constitutes one of the crowning achievements of antibiotics, whose use has been responsible for reducing their number and seriousness. It may even have been too successful for its own good, as the abuse of prescribed antibiotics for treatment of this condition is all too common. Conversely, there is no consistent standard treatment for sore throats of viral origin.

ACUPOINT TREATMENT

For eliminating pain from the throat, acupoint therapy is irreplaceable. Burning sensations, pain, and trouble swallowing are all very quick to disappear under treatment. If the problem is a simple viral sore throat, this treatment can be enough on its own to get rid of it entirely.

TECHNIQUES TO USE

Massage the two principal points with your finger or with an electrical stimulator until a sensation of numbness replaces the burning pain in the throat. Repeat these massages two or three times a day, with a half-hour interval between sessions.

An acute sore throat that is benign should disappear within a day's time. If it does not, consult your physician.

The Principal Points

The first principal point is located on the back of the thumb, outside the corner of the thumbnail, on the edge that is closer to the index finger.

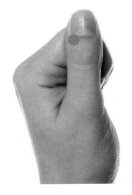 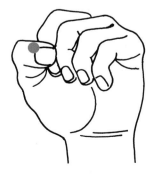

The Principal Points (continued)

The second principal point is one finger-width
behind the corner of the jaw.

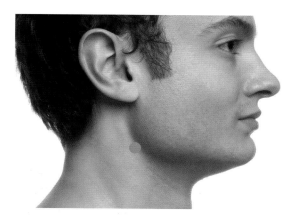
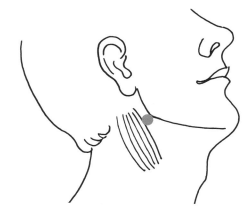

The Secondary Points

The first of these points is found on the back
of the hand in the angle formed by the bones
leading to the thumb and index finger. The
second accessory point is at the end of the
second toe, on the side facing the outer edge
of the foot, in the corner by the bottom end
of the toenail.

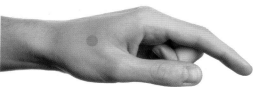
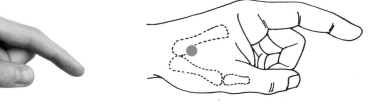

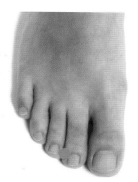
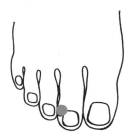

Mumps

A CLASSIC CHILDHOOD disease (but one that can also occur during adulthood), mumps is a virus that attacks the salivary glands and the parotid gland in particular.

SYMPTOMS

In its standard manifestation, this illness is characterized by a deformity first on one side of the face, then both, behind the jaw. It causes this normally bony part of the face to become swollen and in its worst cases can make the shape of the individual's head resemble a pear. This swelling is accompanied by a more or less high fever and sometimes causes the outbreak of a light rash.

Other glands can be afflicted in addition to the parotid gland, which is what makes this disease so potentially serious. It often also targets the genital glands, causing inflammation of one or both testicles in males, or of the ovaries in females. In addition to sharp pains in these organs, mumps contacted after puberty can sometimes cause sterility.

We also know that mumps can attack the pancreas, and is thereby one of the causes of diabetes.

Increasingly, mumps is associated with cases of meningitis in children, though these cases are most often not as serious as they may seem.

STANDARD TREATMENT

Like all diseases caused by viruses, there is no specific treatment for mumps. Only rest, analgesics, and anti-inflammatory medications are used. In cases of orchitis (inflammation of the testicles), the patient must remain confined to bed. Sometimes it is treated with female hormones.

ACUPOINT TREATMENT

Acupoint therapy is recommended for mumps because of its innocuous nature and its rapid action; it is quite capable of reducing pain and swelling, and can also shorten the development time of the disease.

TECHNIQUES TO USE

In most cases, you can massage the points below every half hour. Use vigorous stimulation. A child can even do this himself.

In serious cases, much more intense stimulation—with needles or electricity—is required.

The Principal Point

The principal point is located behind the ear, perpendicular to the parotid gland at the tip of the mastoid bone.

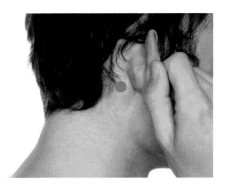

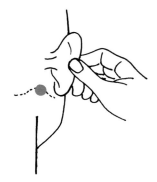

The Secondary Points

The first of the secondary points is located in the center of the wrist on the palmar side, three finger-widths beneath the fold. The second point is at the bottom of the angle formed where the thumb and the index finger meet, against the bone that connects to the index finger.

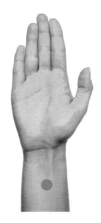

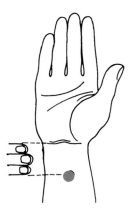

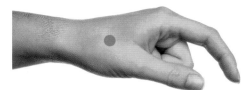

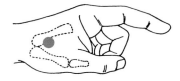

PART TWO

Glands and
Overall Health

Thyroid Disorders:
Goiter and Graves' Disease

THE THYROID GLAND, situated at the base of the throat, is vulnerable to disorders of hyper- and hypoactivity.

Goiter is an increase in the volume of the thyroid gland, causing a concomitant increase in thyroid hormone. When this gland starts functioning too much, it becomes "toxic" and causes problems throughout the body. This state is known as hyperthyroidism.

SYMPTOMS

Simple goiter reveals its presence by a swelling of the throat in front of the Adam's apple. This deformity tends to be irregular—sometimes it is unilateral, at other times it can sink down into the tho-

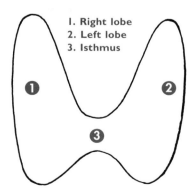

1. Right lobe
2. Left lobe
3. Isthmus

Shape of the thyroid gland

rax below the sternum. The swelling can sometimes achieve enormous size. Simple goiter can remain in the same state for an entire lifetime. It does sometimes continue to slowly increase in size, and may eventually constrict the respiratory tract.

Toxic goiter, on the other hand, is rather on the small side, and is fairly often raised by the beating of the arteries of the neck. It is accompanied by:

- Weight loss
- Palpitations
- A state of high nervousness
- Protrusion of the eyes forward from their orbit—called *exophthalmos*. The eyes can also become shiny.

Toxic goiter can appear in two forms: the thyroid gland can become entirely enveloped, as in the case of Graves' disease, or a part of the thyroid gland—a node—sticks out and becomes palpable in an otherwise normal gland; this is a toxic nodule. Neither form should be allowed to develop unchecked; it will lead to cardiac insufficiency and eventual heart failure. There can also be eye problems caused by exophthalmos.

A medical examination will allow a clear differentiation between the two types of goiter. In simple goiter, everything else is normal. Toxic goiter, on the other hand, will be accompanied by other signs and symptoms:

- Blood tests will reveal a lower cholesterol rate and a pronounced increase of iodine, as well as elevated levels of thyroid hormones.
- The Achilles tendon reflex will react too quickly when stimulated by the percussion of a hammer.
- The gland itself can be injected with a weak dose of radioactive iodine, then scanned to evaluate the location of hyperactivity.

CAUSES

Simple goiter occurs in areas where the diet lacks iodine.

As far as the cause of toxic goiter is concerned, the medical establishment has changed its opinion: originally it was blamed on a harmful effect of the pituitary gland. Now it seems more likely that the thyroid somehow "encases" itself—perhaps under the effect of a virus.

STANDARD TREATMENT

Simple goiter is the province of surgery. For toxic goiter, iodine was originally the standard treatment. This protocol was gradually replaced by a combination of surgery to remove the nodules and radioactive iodine to deactivate the gland. Today, the most common treatments are pharmaceutical products known as "antithyroids," which lower the secretion rate of thyroid hormones.

ACUPOINT TREATMENT

There is little benefit from acupoint therapy in the treatment of simple goiter, but it provides a useful supplement to the use of antithyroid drugs in cases of toxic goiter; it often permits lower dosages to be used. It also relieves the discomforts caused by this disease.

TECHNIQUES TO USE

As we are dealing with a chronic affliction, it is best to stimulate the points for a few minutes at a time, several times a day, or to apply a continuous stimulus for a ten-minute period every other day, for example.

The Points

The first of the points is located on the palm side of the wrist, right in the center, about three finger-widths below the fold where the hand bends. The second point is located along the inner edge of the tibia bone in a small notch, a hand-width above the ankle; the third is located on the edge of the skull, three finger-widths away from the median line.

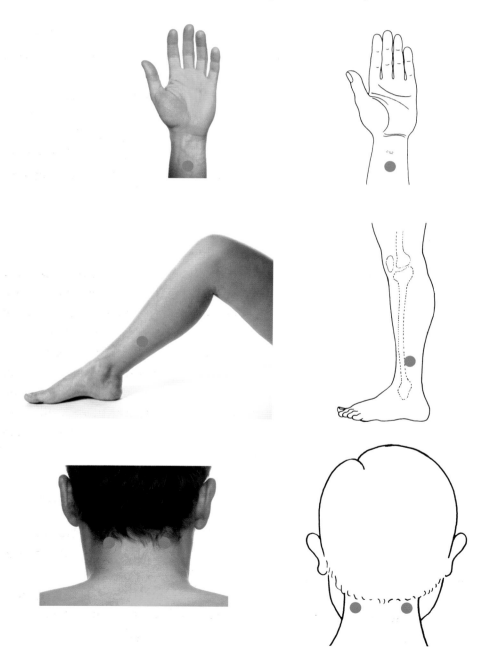

Diabetes

DIABETES MELLITUS IS characterized by excessive sugar in the blood and urine. There are essentially two forms of the disease, or to be more precise, two different diseases:

- Type 1 diabetes (which has replaced the older terms of "juvenile diabetes," "thin diabetes," and so forth) occurs most often in childhood and causes weight loss.
- Type 2 diabetes (formerly known as "obesity-related diabetes," "adult onset diabetes," and so on) occurs primarily among older adults, and is usually accompanied by obesity.

SYMPTOMS

There are three signs that should demand attention: eating too much, drinking too much, and urinating too much.

CAUSES

There is one organ that is solely responsible for both forms of this disease—the pancreas. It releases insulin, a substance that regulates the sugar level in the body. In type 1 diabetes, the pancreas does not release any insulin, while in type 2 diabetes, there may be insufficient quantities of insulin, or it may be poorly used by the body.

We know now that type 1 diabetes is generally not hereditary, contrary to what was long believed. It seems more likely due to the actual destruction of the pancreas by a virus—one such as mumps, for example. On the other hand, type 2 diabetes is a hereditary disease that is quite often linked to obesity, and is preceded by a long pre-diabetic phase.

STANDARD TREATMENT

For type 1 diabetes, the standard treatment is an injection of insulin one or more times a day combined with a very strict diet. Future treatments will undoubtedly include pancreas grafts or implanted insulin pumps.

For type 2 diabetes, the first treatment step is weight loss. If there is no regression of the diabetes despite weight loss, pills will be added to the treatment to lower blood sugar levels.

ACUPOINT TREATMENT

Acupoint therapy is at best an adjuvant procedure in the treatment of diabetes 1 and 2. It is less effective than medication, but can provide helpful reinforcement that may ultimately allow patients to reduce the amount of medication they require.

TECHNIQUES TO USE

As with other chronic conditions, long and repeated stimulation of the points is necessary to produce an effect: massage or electrical stimulation for ten minutes, two to three times a day will support diabetes treatment.

The Points

The first point is located on both sides of the spinal column, a finger-width away from the spine at the level of the bottom of the shoulder blade. The second point is behind the inner ankle, a finger-width below the edge of the calcaneum bone; the third is on the outer surface of the leg, one hand-width below the fold of the knee.

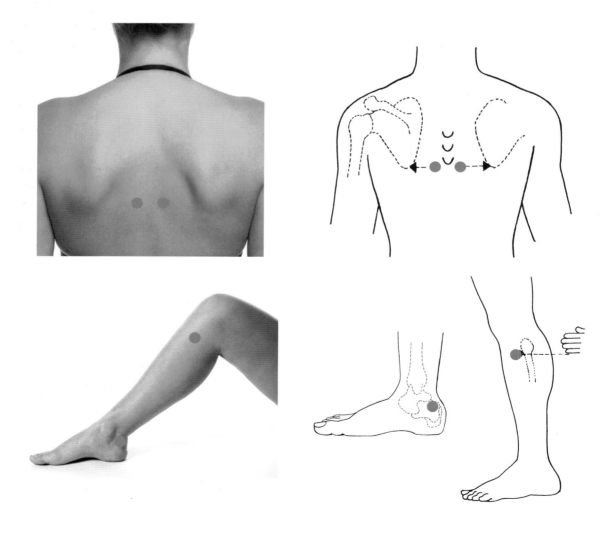

Obesity

BY DEFINITION AN obese individual is a man or woman who is too fat. While this definition has the merit of being simple, it only raises a problem and does not solve it. In fact, at just what point does an individual begin to become obese? And what are the real drawbacks to being too fat?

Of course, it has been shown unequivocally that obesity is correlated with higher rates of certain diseases such as diabetes, heart disease, and kidney disease. So from that perspective, obesity constitutes a hazard to one's health. However, being moderately overweight—about 25 pounds, for example—has not been shown to increase the chance of death from these diseases, and even seems to confer some benefits in protecting people from other ailments.

SYMPTOMS

In this regard, I should mention that there are two kinds of obesity: one is a consequence of illness and the other a consequence of lifestyle. It was American health insurance companies in the 1950s that first raised an alarm about obesity. For crude financial motives, they demonstrated that life expectancy decreased in direct proportion to the amount of excess weight a person carried.

At the same time, Western standards of beauty were changing, influenced by the increased popularity of sporting activities, and the advent of a leisure society in which people now had the liberty to stroll on beaches nearly nude. These changes helped promote the idealized images of flat-bellied men and women with the slender figure of a fashion model. Now, the opulent beauty of the Renaissance and the plump middle-class individuals of the early twentieth century have become objects of repulsion. You have to live in accordance with your times . . .

In modern times, there has been a desire to find a mathematical model for obesity. Methods for calculating obesity have flourished, the best known being Lorentz's formula, according to which the ideal weight is determined by the following:

$$\text{Ideal male weight (in kg)* =}$$
$$\text{Height (in cm)} - 100 - \frac{[\text{height (in cm)} - 150]}{4}$$

$$\text{Ideal female weight (in kg) =}$$
$$\text{Height (in cm)} - 100 - \frac{[\text{height (in cm)} - 150]}{2.5}$$

*Note: 1 kg = 2.2 lbs; 1 inch = 2.54 cm

In truth, it does not seem that any of these formulas offer any absolute validity. It may be better to classify obesity within two broad categories, according to morphological and psychological criteria.

1. Morphological criteria define the "shape" of the body. With this as a guide, we can distinguish: *android obesity,* a typically "male" kind of obesity wherein the overweight is concentrated in the upper part of the body; *gynoid obesity,* which typically affects women, and concentrates excess fat on the lower half of the body; *cellulite,* which are "pockets" of fat confined to individual parts of the body. This is a source of despair for many women on whom these pockets can appear on the thighs, the hips, knees, or ankles.

   Each of these kinds of obesity is accompanied by its own characteristic illnesses and disorders. Android obesity is often partnered by high blood pressure and cardiac disease, while gynoid obesity often appears with vein disorders (varicose veins, phlebitis) in the lower limbs. Cellulite brings along its own baggage of irritants, which are mostly emotional. It often becomes an ongoing source of depression because even losing weight overall does not necessarily get rid of these pockets of fat.

2. Then, we must also take the psychological factors into account. There are many overweight individuals who are happy and flourishing, who feel comfortable with who they are. And if they are only moderately overweight, they may not be subjecting themselves to health risks at all.

There are also people whose weight is not an issue yet who think they are fat, a phenomenon that afflicts women more than men. They live with one eye constantly staring at the needle on the scales. These are people who it is necessary to convince their overweight is a figment of their imagination, no easy task!

Then there are all the rest who really do need to become thinner and whose weight is a source of suffering and health problems. It is these people for whom this chapter is written.

CAUSES

The search for the causes of obesity has been responsible for the expenditure of billions of dollars and for the flow of a lot of ink.

Opinions on this subject have evolved hugely over the years. Initially, obesity was blamed primarily on the "glands," especially because a few rare endocrine diseases (myxedema, for example) were accompanied by excess fat. This turned out to be more the exception than the rule, however. The next culprit was "polyphagia"—a disease of overeating. When Freudian thought was popular in the early twentieth century, obese people were thought to be stuck in an "oral phase." Finally, our own time has turned its sights on heredity and is striving to identify the "genes" responsible for a stout physique.

There is a little truth in each of these theories:

• Hereditary factors often do play a role in obesity, and there are entire families that are overweight. This hereditary factor may be linked to a genetic predisposition toward diabetes, as the two diseases often occur simultaneously.

- Inherited bad habits are at least as common as inherited genes, however. Though they may originate from good faith, bad habits like "forced feeding" begin in infancy and many people eat too much completely unaware that they are doing so.

- Current lifestyles allow people to spend far too much time sitting in their offices or their automobiles, or in front of a computer or television screen, eating overly large meals and snacks of all sorts that quickly contribute to excess weight.

- Some individuals "munch" throughout the day as a compensation for boredom or anxiety.

- And quite recently, there has been the discovery that neurotransmitters—those mysterious messengers of the nervous system—are to blame. In adult obesity, the release of insulin has the effect of loading the cells with fat. Childhood obesity may be triggered by excessive secretion of prolactin, a hormone that is normally "charged" by lactation, which then multiplies the number of fat cells.

STANDARD TREATMENT

The foundation of every treatment is a serious diet, of which there are many. The difficulty is not in losing weight, however, but in keeping it off, which is made all the more challenging by the lives we lead today. What can be done to help keep this weight off?

Although many people dream of a medication that would help them grow thinner, there are very few drugs that actually achieve this goal. Let's speak first of all the ones that should be avoided: appetite suppressants, thyroidal extracts, and diuretics. The first are dangerous for the nerves and the other two are not logical prescriptions for obesity as neither the thyroid gland nor water are to blame. What then remains? There are a few medications that are sometimes prescribed for morbidly obese people who are unable to lose weight in other ways. However, these can have serious side effects, and patients typically re-gain weight once they stop taking the drugs.

ACUPOINT TREATMENT

The classic Chinese authors showed next to no interest in obesity, as fat was a sign of social success. However, considerable efforts have been made in the past several years to determine more precise points that have an effect on appetite. They work very well for some people and are well worth trying for that reason, but they are not effective for everyone.

TECHNIQUES TO USE

It is necessary to stimulate these points twenty minutes by hand or ten minutes electrically, at least twice a day. When used in conjunction with dieting, the results are often excellent.

The Points

There are two points on the body, and two on the ear. The first point is found on the outer side of the calf, a hand-width beneath the fold of the knee when it is bent. The second point is located on the side of the torso, on the inner edge of the thorax at the tip of the last (floating) rib.

The first point on the ear is one millimeter in front of the inner extremity of the tragus, the little "bump" located in front of the ear; the second is the little "bump" at the top of the earlobe.

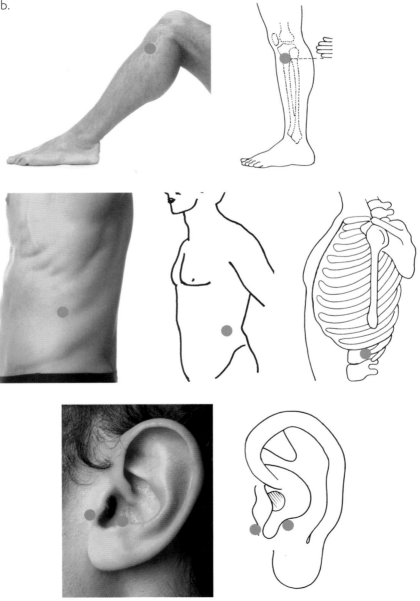

PART THREE

Rheumatology

Arthritis

THERE ARE TWO major forms of arthritis: osteoarthritis and rheumatoid arthritis. Osteoarthritis is an erosive and degenerative form of the condition. The cartilage that covers joints becomes worn away and disappears, causing the bones to rub together— severely—therefore causing pain and deformity. This can occur with joints in the vertebrae, the hips, the knees, the fingers, the toes, and so forth.

The onset of osteoarthritis normally begins later in life, starting usually after an individual's fiftieth birthday. The causes of osteoarthritis are still a mystery, although "wear and tear" on the joints is certainly a factor. Personally, I believe that osteoarthritis is almost always a complication of an articular displacement, in other words, a situation in which the joints or the bones are no longer in their proper place. This displacement, which is obvious when it occurs in the hip, for example, may be less obvious in other joints.

Rheumatoid arthritis, on the other hand, is an infection or inflammation inside the joint and the fluid that lubricates it. This fluid, the synovial fluid, is held in a small fibrous sac inside the joint. There are a variety of causes of rheumatoid arthritis that can be viral or bacterial in origin; most often the disease will occur in hereditarily predisposed terrain.

Some forms of arthritis attack the spinal column causing it to become fixed and stiff; others primarily strike the elbows, knees, wrists, fingers, and so forth, causing them to become deformed.

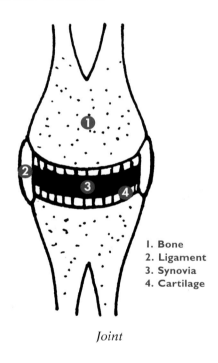

1. Bone
2. Ligament
3. Synovia
4. Cartilage

Joint

STANDARD TREATMENT

Despite the diversity of their causes, the treatment of the different forms of arthritis almost always includes the same prescription: rest, and general or local anti-inflammatory medications, including injections of cortisone. However, continued use of these medications can be dangerous, particularly for the stomach.

ACUPOINT TREATMENT

The stimulation of the points is effective for arthritis in part because of the therapy's analgesic effect. But acupoint therapy also works against swelling and redness. During acupuncture, one can often watch the inflammation decrease during treatment. Therefore, acupoint treatment is always indicated for arthritic conditions because of its effectiveness and its innocuous nature.

As much as possible, it is helpful to treat the stricken joint itself, by stimulating points that specifically address it. Throughout this part of the book, I will therefore describe points that best treat the different areas of the body most often afflicted by arthritic and rheumatic conditions.

However, when a large number of joints are affected, for example by severe polyarthritis, or a wide-spread case of osteoarthritis, when the individual's body seems positively rotten with rheumatism, with multiple sources of pain all over the body, general points may be the most effective.

TECHNIQUES TO USE

When dealing with chronic pain, it is necessary to stimulate these points two or three times a day using massage or electricity.

In an acute outburst, the session should be shorter. The massages will be more superficial and not as deep.

The Points

For arthritis in general, the first point is located on the lower edge of the inner ankle bone, in the small notch on the front edge of the bone, in the crease that is formed when standing.

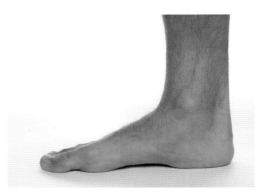
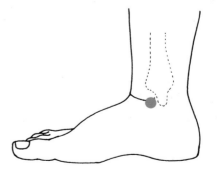

The Points (continued)

The second point is on the nape of the neck, two finger-widths away on either side of the first visible protrusion—the seventh cervical vertebra. These points can be found most easily by bending the head slightly forward.

The third point is on the back of the forearm, halfway between either side and at the midpoint between the wrist crease and the elbow crease.

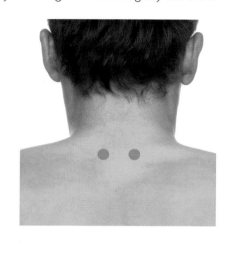

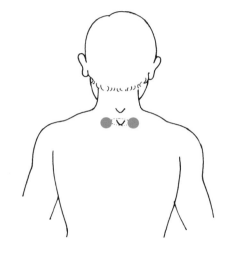

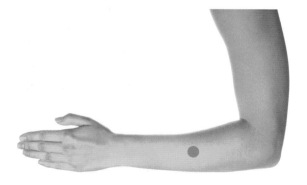

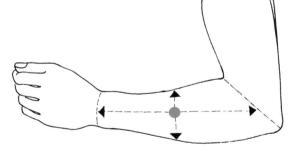

Stiff Neck

A STIFF NECK is an acute problem arising from a blockage in the neck. Other pains in the area can be more or less chronic.

The symptoms of most neck disorders are well-known. As the result of an awkward movement or simply from sleeping in a poor position, the neck feels taut. Sometimes, it is impossible to turn your head.

CAUSES

There are some serious afflictions that can affect the vertebrae of the neck, including tumors, infections, and arthritis. Caution is the watchword here when a traumatic injury is the cause, because there may be a vertebral fracture (especially after an automobile accident). This is why an x-ray is always called for in the event of an injury like this.

But in the vast majority of cases, we are dealing with the displacement of one or more vertebrae. This can occur as the result of a shock or from having assumed a poor position repeatedly; the vertebrae slide over one another blocking the nerves that pass between them.

Some cases of neck pain are caused by osteoarthritis. It could be said that vertebral osteoarthritis is not painful by itself; what causes the pain is the constriction of nerves between the twisted vertebrae. This is the major cause of all the health problems in this area of the body.

Nerve constriction will first cause a localized pain, followed by muscle contractions in the neck. If one of the upper cervical vertebrae is primarily affected, it can also cause migraines or other types of headache.

If, on the contrary, one of the lower cervical vertebrae is affected, the pains will descend into the shoulder and down the arm, sometimes even reaching the hand. This condition is then a cervical brachial neuralgia, more simply called "neuritis."

In all cases, dizzy spells can also occur. Cervical displacement is one of the most frequent causes of vertigo because the vertebral artery that goes into the cerebellum—the center of balance—travels through the cervical vertebrae and can easily be pinched.

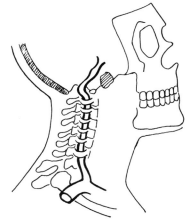

The vertebral artery passes through the cervical column.

STANDARD TREATMENT

Standard treatment for neck pain consists of sedatives and muscle relaxants, which treat the symptoms and not the cause. A very effective treatment for stiff neck and other neck pain is vertebral manipulation, which puts the bones that have been displaced back in their proper locations. But a manipulation of this nature should be performed by a highly trained osteopath or chiropractor, once other causes of a more serious nature such as fractures or tumors have been eliminated.

ACUPOINT TREATMENT

The role played here by acupoint therapy is extremely important, and I can safely say that stimulation of these points not only makes it possible to avoid the use of any pain medications but can even, by reducing the muscle contractions, contribute to the spontaneous return of the vertebrae to their proper position.

TECHNIQUES TO USE

As with all acute disorders, you should vigorously stimulate the appropriate point or points until the pain subsides, and repeat the treatment as often as necessary. This stimulation can be performed either manually or electrically.

The Principal Point

The principal point is located on the edge of the hand below the little finger, on the heart line next to the bone that connects to the finger.

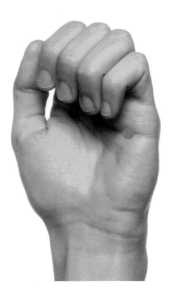

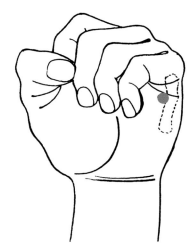

The Secondary Points

The first of the secondary points is located two finger-widths above the middle of the calf on its outer edge; the second point is on the back of the hand between the index and middle fingers.

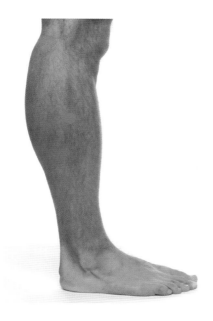

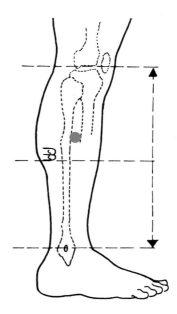

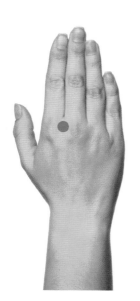

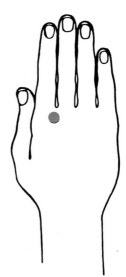

Shoulder Pain:
Cervical Brachial Neuralgia

CERVICAL BRACHIAL NEURALGIA is an irritation of the nerve that runs through the arm and the shoulder. There is generally no restriction of movement, but an aching sensation runs from the neck to the hand. The pain appears along the course of the nerve, and at its maximum severity, affects the entire arm from the neck to the hand. It has the nature of a nerve pain—sometimes burning, sometimes stabbing or tingling. Effective treatment depends in part on being able to map out the exact course of the pain.

CAUSES

Cervical bracial neuralgia is generally caused by the constriction of one or more nerves at their roots. In the vast majority of cases, this nerve constriction is due to the displacement of one or more of the cervical vertebrae from osteoarthritis.

This kind of neuralgia can clear up on its own if the ribs return spontaneously to their normal position. But in the majority of cases, this return takes place in a manner that is both imperfect and slow.

STANDARD TREATMENT

The main treatment offered for cervical brachial neuralgia relies on sedatives and anti-inflammatory drugs. Sometimes these are accompanied by a neck manipulation that restores the vertebrae to their proper places and un-jams the nerves.

ACUPOINT TREATMENT

Acupoint therapy soothes the pain and removes the muscular contraction that is often associated with this kind of neuralgia. It can suffice on its own to restore the body to order. In any event, it is always a valuable reinforcement for other treatments.

TECHNIQUES TO USE

Because this is an acute disorder, it is appropriate to stimulate the points strongly starting at the time the pain appears and continuing until it subsides. Repeat as often as necessary.

The Points

The treatment called for here brings into play one of the most ancient rules of Chinese medicine: the use of the meridian. For effective treatment, the exact course of the pain should be identified. Roughly speaking, these courses are three in number and can terminate in one of three places:

1. The side of the thumb
2. Toward the middle of the back of the hand
3. The side of the little finger

The points are then located at the top and bottom of the appropriate finger. Even if the actual pain stops at some point further up on the arm, it should be followed to where it would naturally end in the corresponding finger, and the points on that finger are the ones that need to be stimulated.

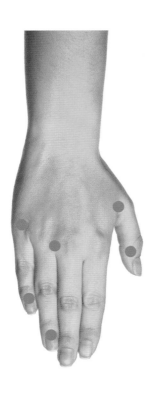

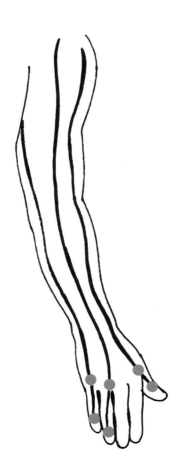

Shoulder Pain:
Periarthritis

PERIARTHRITIS REFERS TO an inflammation of one or both of the joints in the shoulder area.

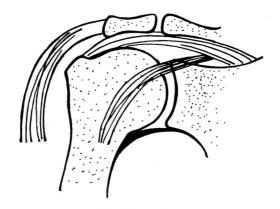

Shoulder joint

Around the joint of the shoulder itself, which is to say the articulation between the humerus (or arm bone) and the shoulder blade, there is essentially a second joint formed by the muscles that surround the shoulder and allow the arm to make all its movements. These muscles operate by means of fluid-filled pockets that are called synovial sacs; they are kind of like ball bearings, as the diagram shows.

SYMPTOMS

The essential sign of periarthritis is the blockage of movement. This blockage can be total—in which case the condition is referred to as "frozen shoulder"—or partial, and felt predominantly in one of the arm's movements, such as scratching the back. The pain makes its presence known when one can no longer complete this movement.

CAUSES

While arthritis may rarely be caused by an infection or a tumor, it is most often a result of inflammation in the tendons or their associated bursa. The inflammation can be caused by the "wear-and-tear" of repetitive motion, by mineral deposits in the joint, or by a direct injury to the area.

STANDARD TREATMENT

The general treatment for shoulder arthritis is rest and anti-inflammatory drugs, then a reeducation of the shoulder by a physical therapist. The most commonly used drug is a cortisone injection directly into the shoulder. But this often has serious risks and can only be repeated two or three times.

ACUPOINT TREATMENT

Acupoint therapy can be quite effective for both the pain and the stiffness of arthritis. It is an excellent idea to combine this treatment with that of a passive or active manipulation of the shoulder by a professional body worker like a physical therapist.

TECHNIQUES TO USE

The points can be stimulated by massage or by electric current. In either case, a long period of stimulation is best—five to ten minutes. Various shoulder movements should be performed during acupoint stimulation: elevate the shoulder toward the front, toward the side, and toward the back, for example. These joint mobilizations will contribute to the pain relief, and greatly improve the range of motion with each session.

The Principal Point

The principal point should be stimulated in all cases. It is located on the front of the shoulder, and can be found in the small hollow that forms there when you hold your arm out straight with the thumb extended upward.

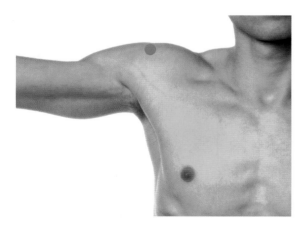
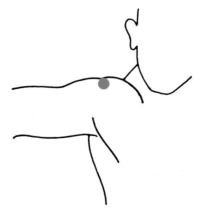

The Secondary Points

The secondary points can be added according to the location of the pain and stiffness. If the front of the shoulder is affected, stimulate the point halfway between the armpit and the principal point described above. If the pain is primarily on the side of the shoulder, stimulate the point directly beneath the tip of the shoulder blade. If the pain and stiffness are on the back of the shoulder, stimulate the point that is located one finger-width above the back edge of the crease of the armpit.

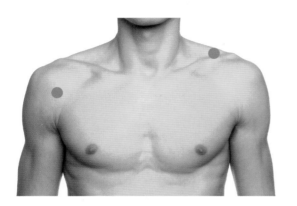
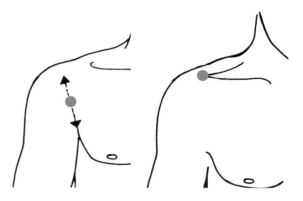

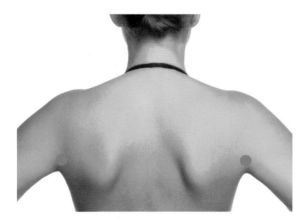
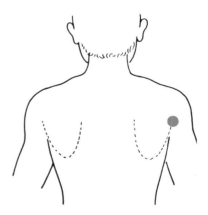

Elbow Pain

THE ELBOW IS composed of four distinct units. There is the elbow joint itself, which contains the joint between the humerus (the upper arm bone), and the bones of the forearm—the radius and the ulna. Then there is a second joint between the two bones of the forearm, located below the elbow crease on the thumb side of the forearm.

Finally, and let me give this special emphasis, there are two false joints. They are located at the end of the humerus bone on two bony spurs that bear the ungracious names of the lateral (little finger side) and medial (thumb side) epicondyles.

An incredible number of muscles are attached to these two prominent spurs—the muscles that allow the hand to move. In fact, there is a veritable tangle here of muscles, tendons, and lubricating pockets, better known by their scientific name of synovial sacs.

Any or all of these muscles, joints, and tendons can become inflamed, especially on the thumb side, causing what is clinically defined as an epicondylitis but is better known as "tennis elbow" because it strikes these athletes disproportionately. But tennis players are not the only ones to be afflicted by it: golfers or even players of a milder sport like bocci ball can suffer from it, as well as anyone whose job requires repetitive gestures. Basket-makers, switchboard operators,

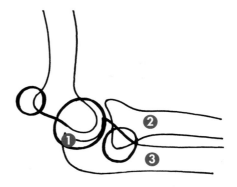

1. Olecranon (part of the ulna bone located behind the humerus)
2. Radius
3. Ulna
4. Humerus

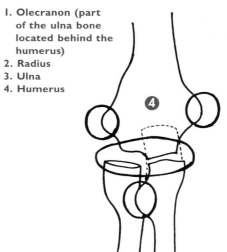

The four "joints" of the elbow

and housewives who often carry heavy bags or baskets can also be affected. The pain will only occur during certain movements, like turning the crank to open a window, for example, but it may become so acute as to prevent many activities.

CAUSES

Elbow pains are typically the result of repetitive strain on the joints and muscles. They can also be caused by direct injury to the area, however, or even an irritation of the nerves.

The condition often evolves over time, sometimes leading to significant pain and disability that can be a catastrophe for the individual's professional life.

STANDARD TREATMENT

As in other arthritic conditions, the standard treatment relies on analgesics and anti-inflammatory drugs, particularly repeated cortisone injections. However, these can literally destroy the muscles and tendons.

ACUPOINT TREATMENT

As with many other pain disorders, acupoint therapy is quite effective with elbow pain, and poses no danger.

TECHNIQUES TO USE

With all pain conditions, the points should be stimulated strongly with massage or electricity until the pain subsides. The Chinese even inject substances with a sedative effect at these points.

In chronic cases, like epicondolytis for example, five- to ten-minute stimulations should be performed two to three times a day, combined with movements of the joint.

The Principal Point

The principal point is located at the outer end of the crease of the elbow, on the thumb side of the arm.

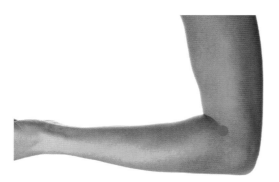
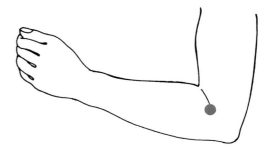

Acupuncture
August 4 | 1 p.m.

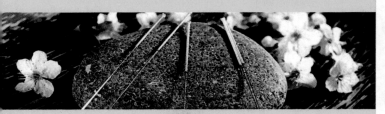

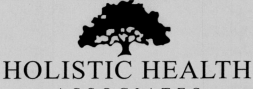

HOLISTIC HEALTH
ASSOCIATES

Join Ryan Diener with Holistic Health as he discusses the benefits of Acupuncture in "The Good Life- An Annual Health Plan"

FREDERICK
COUNTY
PUBLIC
LIBRARIES

Walkersville Branch
2 South Glade Road
Walkersville, MD
301-600-8200

fcpl.org

The Secondary Points

There are two secondary points: One is three finger-widths below the preceding point, on the edge of the forearm; the other is on the back of the hand, at the bottom of the space separating the thumb from the index finger. The point is located against the bone of the index finger, near its end.

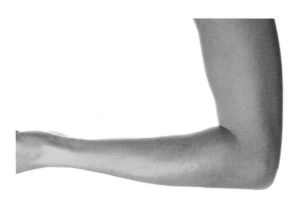 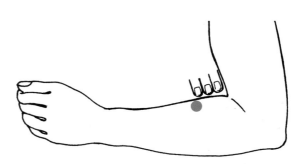

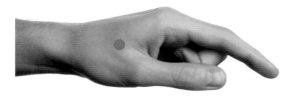 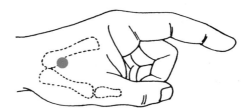

Wrist Pain

THE WRIST JOINT consists of fifteen bones in all (the two bones of the forearm—the radius and the ulna, the eight small bones of the wrist, and the five metacarpal bones that connect with the finger bones). This bone group forms the floor of a kind of room, whose ceiling is formed by a single large ligament, the ring finger ligament of the carpus. Extending through this room are the tendons and nerves connecting to the fingers.

SYMPTOMS AND FORMS

There are two very different causes for wrist pain. In one, arthritis attacks the wrist joint, often as part of an inflammatory disease like polyarthritis. It is painful and causes swelling and deformity of the affected area. The other disorder is carpal tunnel syndrome, whose symptoms are sensations of pain, numbness, or tingling in the palm or wrist. Sometimes, particularly at night, the individual will experience a burning sensation in the hand and fingers. Women are frequently the victims of this affliction during menopause.

STANDARD TREATMENT

General treatments using anti-inflammatory drugs are used for arthritis of the wrist.

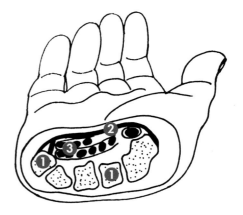

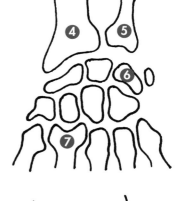

1. The bones
2. Transverse carpal ligament
3. Tendons and their sheath
4. Radius
5. Ulna
6. Carpal bones
7. Metacarpal bones (these are the bones that connect to the finger bones and make up the palm of the hand)
8. Transverse ligament in the skin

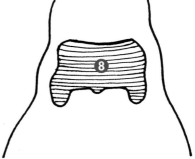

Anatomy of the wrist

Carpal tunnel syndrome is treated initially by injections of cortisone. If the cortisone does not seem to be working, surgery is generally the next option. The operation uses a section of the wrist ligament.

ACUPOINT TREATMENT

Pressure point therapy is very helpful for treating wrist arthritis as it reduces pain and inflammation. It is also a valuable treatment option for carpal tunnel syndrome as it can allow the patient to avoid the more aggressive standard treatments involving steroids and surgery.

TECHNIQUES TO USE

Stimulate the points in accordance with the general rule for this kind of disorder: in cases of acute pain, massage the point until the pain disappears. For chronic pain, two or three massages per day for several minutes each time are called for. These massages, especially for carpal tunnel syndrome, should be deep and prolonged until there is a tingling sensation in the hand. This kind of stimulation is much easier to perform using an electrical device.

The Principal Points

The first point is located on the back of the hand, two finger-widths below the crease of the wrist, between the two bones of the forearm.

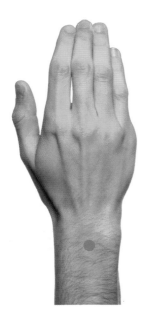
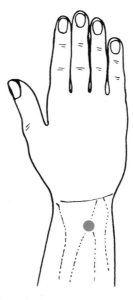

The Principal Points (continued)

The second point is on the palmar side of the wrist, at the edge of the crease that is nearest the pinkie finger.

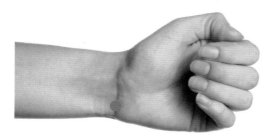

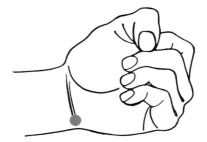

The Secondary Point

There is one additional point for treating carpal tunnel syndrome: it is located at the very center of the wrist crease on the palm side. It should be massaged quite deeply using great force, going all the way to the bone.

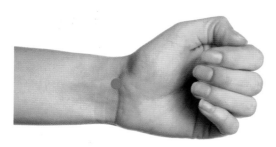

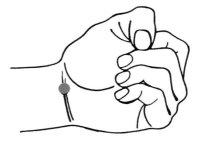

Finger Pain

THE FINGERS ARE probably the least protected part of our bodies and can often fall victim to trauma or infection.

Any disorder affecting the fingers should be addressed quickly because it can, if left untreated, seriously affect the more complex structures like the tendons, joints, and bones. A simple finger infection can lead to disaster if left untreated. The same holds true for bites and stings, as the tiny entry door they create can lead to enormous damage in the depths of the body.

But among the most common problems affecting the fingers is rheumatism, which here, too, occurs in two major varieties:

- In inflammatory rheumatism, the fingers are the site of choice for polyarthritis, which can cause them to curl up like claws.
- Degenerative forms of rheumatism, otherwise known as osteoarthritis, can be particularly severe during menopause. The fingers become deformed in this situation as well, but in a different manner: nodes appear that are quite painful, especially during the time they are forming. The base of the thumb is particularly affected.

In both cases, these afflictions can cause considerable problems for the many move-

ments our fingers are expected to perform. The discomfort will first appear during fine movements such as knitting or writing, then

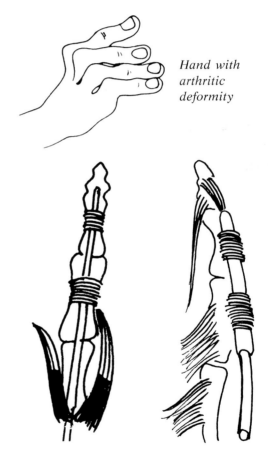

Hand with arthritic deformity

View of the finger beneath the skin seen from the front and in profile. Here we can see all the bones, tendons, sheaths, and ligaments, which makes it easy to grasp just what kind of extensive damage this affliction can cause.

little by little, the hand will lose its strength and start dropping things.

STANDARD TREATMENT

In addition to the basic anti-inflammatory drugs, pharmaceutical medicine suggests local injections of cortisone. These injections are quite painful and difficult when delivered into the small joints of the fingers.

ACUPOINT TREATMENT

Acupoint therapy provides good results and can always be tried first, before resorting to the more problematic standard treatments.

TECHNIQUES TO USE

Massage the points with vigor until the acute pain subsides. For chronic afflictions, stimulate the points two or three times a day for several minutes at a time.

The Points

The principal point is located on the back of each finger, in the middle of the first finger joint (the one located closest to the hand). If several fingers are affected, these points should be stimulated in the following order: **1.** ring finger **2.** thumb **3.** middle finger **4.** index finger **5.** little finger. Of course other points can also be massaged on the other finger joints, or at the base of the fingers, if necessary.

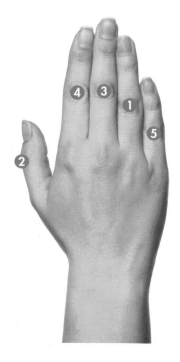

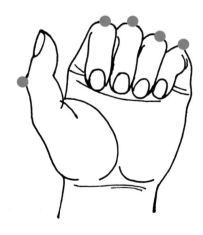

Back Pain

"I HAVE A pain in my back." This is the complaint of typists, mechanical draftsmen, dentists, pianists, and all those who generally work sitting down and leaning forward. This position causes pain, which can affect the spinal column anywhere between the nape of the neck and the region of the kidneys.

Back pain generally involves a dull, stabbing pain, whose onset is commonly in the evening after work hours. More rarely, it manifests in the form of an acute pain after exertion (like lifting up a heavy piece of furniture). This is a more severe kind of lower back pain, which is similar to stiff neck or to the lumbago that affects the lumbar region. But it is much rarer.

CAUSES

The causes are always the same when dealing with the vertebral column: the shifting of a rib, which pinches the roots of a nerve causing contraction and pain along its course.

The nerves that originate in the upper thoracic vertebrae are known as the intercostal nerves. Any intercostal nerve pain or a stitch in the side can thus be the sign of a dorsal misalignment. On the other hand, the nerves originating in the lower spinal column are beneath the skin of the stomach, and the pain they cause can be mistaken as the symptom of a problem in the liver and/or stomach.

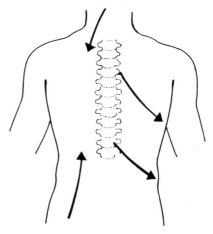

Two false dorsal pains whose actual origins are cervical and lumbar

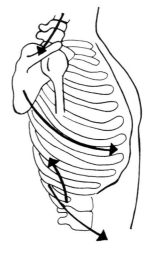

Two types of radiating pain: intercostal and abdominal

Sometimes back pain can actually originate in the nape of the neck, causing pain in the back by way of the nerves that go up and down the spinal column. This is the case for typists whose pain starts from the nape of the neck.

STANDARD TREATMENT

The medical profession bases their treatment on rest, analgesics, and sometimes cortisone shots. But a vertebral manipulation is the most logical treatment to prescribe here, as long as it's performed by a competent chiropractor or other health professional. This will restore the vertebrae to their proper places and eliminate the pain at its source.

ACUPOINT TREATMENT

Acupoint therapy is always very helpful for back pain. In addition to alleviating the pain, it reduces the muscle contractions, and makes manipulation of the area much easier.

TECHNIQUES TO USE

Stimulate the points vigorously in cases of acute pain, until the pain disappears. To prevent and provide relief to those with chronic back problems, stimulate the point for ten minutes in the morning and ten minutes in the evening.

The Point

There is one extremely important point located on the back of the hand, in the corner of the space separating the ring finger and the little finger.

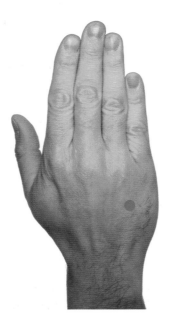 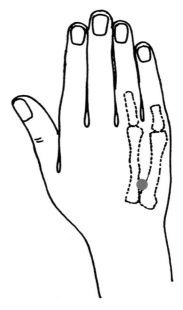

Low Back Pain and Other Problems of the Lumbar Region

MANY PEOPLE COMPLAIN today about kidney pain. In reality, their kidneys have nothing to do with it. This pain is related to a disorder affecting the lower vertebral column, also called the lumbar region.

The most common signs of disturbances in the spinal column are pain and limited movement. In cases involving the lumbar spine, the pain is located on one or the other side of the spinal column, and descends more or less to the buttocks. The seriousness of the condition can range from simple lumbar pain to lumbo-sciatica, which can go all the way down into the feet.

The limitation of movement is obvious. The sufferer may be unable to stoop down, tie his shoes, and so forth, or to the contrary, may be unable to get back up after doing so. The spine may be visibly twisted toward one direction or another.

FORMS

This health problem can start at a very young age, usually as the result of making an effort when in an awkward position. The person may have been trying to pick something up or move a heavy object, during which they experienced a sharp pain "in the kidneys," like being stabbed by a knife. Afterward, movement may have been constricted. This is acute lumbago, otherwise known as a back sprain.

The patient is immobilized and cannot put one foot in front of the other. This condition may last for several days, even several weeks. Then either spontaneously or in response to treatment, things will gradually return to normal.

But far too often the problem resurfaces and the individual finds himself immobile again in a few weeks or months. Repeated bouts of acute low back pain will turn the individual into a chronic sufferer who is constantly in pain—especially in the morning—and whose back will lock up from time to time.

Another drawback of these outbreaks that many people fail to take into account is the economic damage they cause. These disorders are one of the greatest reasons for work absences and have an adverse effect on productivity.

CAUSES

You could say that "back pain" is an illness specific to our civilization, in which few people get all the exercise they need. People go from the bed to the elevator to their car or the subway, and from there to a desk or an assembly line.

To truly grasp the mechanics of low back pain, you have to keep in mind the structure of the vertebral column at the lumbar level. The vertebrae are connected to each other by means of discs, which separate them and act like a kind of shock absorber. These discs consist of a rigid outer surface and a gelatinous core. When a disc herniates—which is the primary cause of low back pain—the semiliquid core spurts through a tear in the sheath, constricting the root of the nerve, and thereby causing pain.

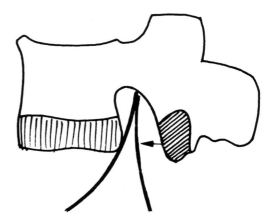

Articular displacement

STANDARD TREATMENT

The standard treatment consists of rest and sedatives. The patient is confined to bed, and sometimes even placed in a cast. Sedatives and muscle relaxants will be combined either as an overall treatment or a local one, in which case it will include cortisone shots. Here again, a skillful spinal manipulation will quite often restore the body to its proper state and eliminate the pain.

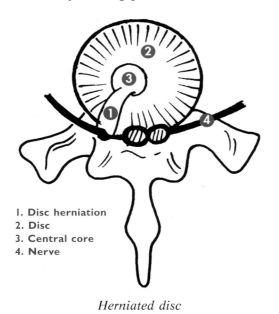

1. **Disc herniation**
2. **Disc**
3. **Central core**
4. **Nerve**

Herniated disc

Another possible cause of acute low back pain, however, can be a sprained rib. One vertebra will shift in position toward another and its back part, the articular apophysis, will pinch the nerve.

ACUPOINT TREATMENT

As in all the other disorders discussed in this section, acupoint therapy can be quite valuable: it calms the pain and reduces the contraction of the muscles.

TECHNIQUES TO USE

Stimulate the points intensely to treat acute low back pain, using massage or electricity. Have the patient try to stand up during the stimulation, which may last from ten to twenty minutes at a time. Sessions can be repeated once an hour. For more chronic pains, sessions of ten to fifteen minutes in the morning and in the evening are called for.

The Principal Point

There is one extremely important point, which is located in the very center of the knee crease, on the back of the knee.

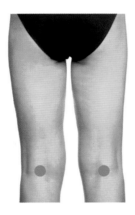 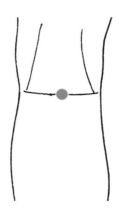

The Secondary Points

One of these is located at the middle of the upper lip beneath the tip of the nose. The other secondary point is found two finger-widths behind the tip of the inner ankle on a small bony bulge.

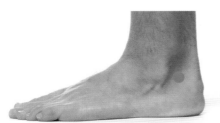 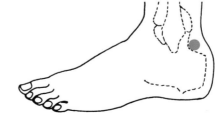

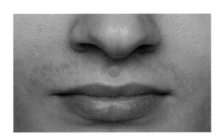 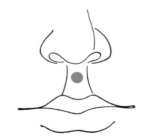

Sciatica

PAIN THAT APPEARS along the path of the sciatic nerve can manifest as burning or stabbing pain, tingling sensations, or numbness—all characteristic of any nerve pain.

But because the sciatic nerve is also a motor nerve that makes the leg move and walk, this motor function can also be affected. Patients may find themselves confronted by a paralyzing case of sciatica that worsens over time, in which the affected limb becomes limp and powerless.

FORMS

In addition to this twofold attack of a sensory and motor nature, the pain can extend to different areas along the entire nerve. For example, one patient may only suffer pain in the buttock or thigh, while another may feel it only in the calf or foot.

It is extremely important to emphasize here the two terminal branches of this nerve: one goes toward the big toe and the other toward the little toe. This therefore gives us two different kinds of sciatica, and two different strategies for treatment.

In fact, the sciatic nerve, which is the longest and thickest nerve in the body, originates from two sets of superimposed nerve roots. For example, when sciatica strikes the big toe, the nerve root that is involved is the one that passes through the fourth and fifth lumbar vertebrae. When it affects the little toe, the nerve root is the one that passes between the fifth lumbar vertebra and the sacral bone. This is of great importance in determining the appropriate treatment.

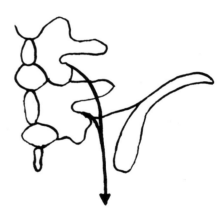

The two roots of the sciatic nerve

CAUSES

Outside of exceptional cases such as tumors or infections, the primary cause of sciatica is still a hot topic of debate. It is often the result of exertion performed with poor posture (lifting a heavy weight for example), or can simply be caused by a coughing fit or a missed step. Once considered to be uniquely due to the result of a herniated disc (the small pad that separates the ribs and can constrict the root),

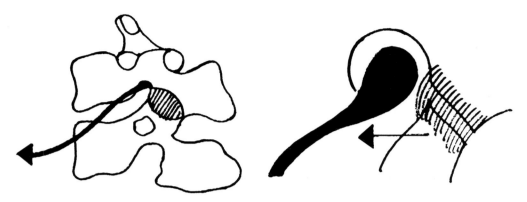

Relative position of the nerve and the vertebrae. It is not hard to see how once this or that rib has shifted place how "easy" it is for the nerve to be pinched: this can be caused by a "slipped" (or herniated) disc, or by the displacement or partial dislocation of one of the vertebra against another.

it now appears that the majority of cases are caused by the displacement of one vertebra against another, which pinches the nerve and causes pain, paralysis, and so on.

If left without treatment, sciatica can continue to make itself known by short and tolerable bursts of pain. But it can also last for weeks, even months, immobilizing the unfortunate sufferer and putting him or her through the worst kind of torture. Little by little the pain will subside, but often a sore spot or numbness remains, for example, in the foot, and the sciatica will return whenever the individual performs any activities requiring exertion.

STANDARD TREATMENT

The best treatment standard medicine has to offer is passive. It can be summed up as follows: bed rest, anesthesia, cortisone shots, and sedatives—which add up to days of pain and work absences. Surgery is often suggested as a last resort, but it does not always provide any lasting solution. In truth, all of this can be avoided and the problem taken care of in very short order by a good vertebral manipulation.

ACUPOINT TREATMENT

Stimulating acupoints can have quite a remarkable effect because in addition to the relaxation it induces both locally and over the entire body, it treats the nerve pain directly.

TECHNIQUES TO USE

Because this is primarily an acute condition, it is necessary to massage the points strongly until the pain subsides. Do this as many times as necessary. If pain persists, then electric stimulation is called for.

The Principal Point

The principal point is one that needs to be stimulated in all cases of sciatica. It is located on the buttock behind the upper end of the femur. In order to find it easily, have the patient stretch out on his healthy side. Spread your fingers and place your hand on the buttock with your thumb along the iliac crest (this is the bony crest at the upper end of the pelvis). Your little finger will be on this point behind the femur.

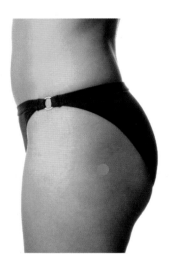

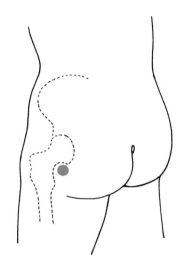

The Secondary Points

The secondary points involve the application of an old Chinese rule that calls for stimulation of the terminal points of the meridians. Where these points are depends on which branch of the nerve is afflicted: if the symptoms concern the branch that goes to the big toe, these points are located at the end of the big toe—one at the bottom edge of the toenail, the other beneath it at the base of the toe. If the symptoms involve the nerve that goes to the little toe, the points are similarly located on the little toe—one at the bottom edge of the toenail, the other beneath it at the base of the toe.

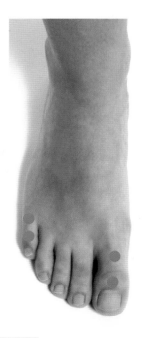

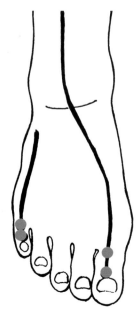

Hip Disorders

THIS CHAPTER CONCERNS anything that can adversely affect the hip joint, the largest and most solid articulation of the body. This joint is responsible for both transmitting and portioning out the weight of the body toward the legs, and for assuring the integrity of one's ability to walk.

A joint with so many responsibilities should have an impeccable structure, but in fact the hip joint is vulnerable to a variety of maladies. It can be attacked by all the health problems that affect the other joints, such as rheumatism, fractures, and so forth, but the most frequent cause of hip impairment is connected with deformities of the joint.

If we take a closer look at the hip we shall see that it in fact forms a kind of key: the top of the femur (the thighbone) fits into a keyhole—the socket of the pelvis. The sad truth is that this key is often almost too large, and the keyhole is just barely big enough. If any deformity exists here—even the smallest impairment—it will cause friction and warping in the joint. The cartilage will deteriorate and this will lead to the most common hip disorder: osteoarthritis of the hip.

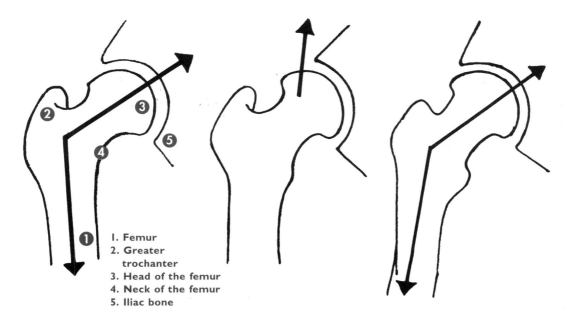

1. Femur
2. Greater trochanter
3. Head of the femur
4. Neck of the femur
5. Iliac bone

Normal hip with a good axis (left); poor covering of the femoral head (center); poor axis, abnormal hips (right)

SYMPTOMS

There are essentially two different symptoms: the first to appear is pain, but it is not always felt at 7the hip itself; it can often radiate to the knee. The next symptom is limping. This is obvious in adults but it has to be carefully examined in children, who have a tendency to conceal this impairment by changing the way they walk. Radiology makes it possible to identify any problems with precision.

STANDARD TREATMENT

The most effective treatment for hip pain is prevention. Starting at birth, efforts should be made to place the bones in a good position by putting a small cushion between the legs of the newborn.

When the damage is too far advanced, only surgery can repair it. The most effective is a complete hip replacement. But many surgeons strive to delay this eventuality for as long as possible. For this reason, they are very receptive to treatment methods that allow them to defer this operation—physical therapy, pain relievers, and so on.

ACUPOINT TREATMENT

Acupoint therapy can be used on its own or in combination with other methods. It is helpful for pain, and can be used without the slightest risk.

TECHNIQUES TO USE

The Chinese sometimes inject calming substances at these points, but massage or electrical stimulation will also be effective.

As always for treatment of pain, two different techniques need to be used, which complement each other perfectly. First, stimulate the point strongly until the pain subsides; then regularly massage the points for fifteen minutes once in the morning and once in the evening, to prevent any acute flare-ups.

The Principal Point

The principal point is located behind the large bone of the hip. Place your thumb on the iliac crest that forms the boundary of the pelvis on the side. Fan your hand out from there over the buttock and your little finger will indicate this point.

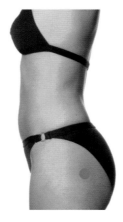
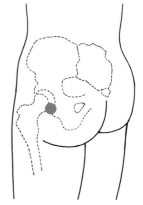

The Secondary Points

The two secondary points can be combined to great advantage: one is right in the middle of the inguinal groove; the other is on the inner side of the leg, a hand-width below the knee at the corner of the tibia bone beneath the kneecap.

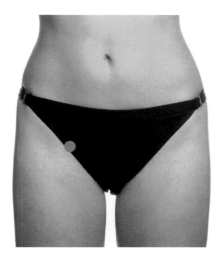

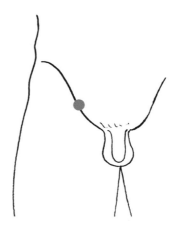

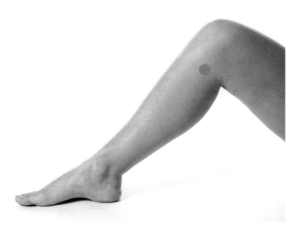

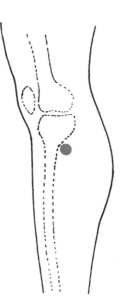

Knee Disorders

THE KNEE IS formed by three bones: the femur, the tibia, and the patella.

Traumatic injury to the knee can cause damage ranging from simple contusions to fractures—including ligament sprains or tears, which are often more serious than the fractures. Certain sports, like soccer, football and skiing, multiply the likelihood of this kind of injury.

Many knee problems are caused by disease. The various forms of arthritis often affect this part of the body, including gout, rheumatoid arthritis, and especially osteoarthritis, which can warp and deform the knees.

Children and adolescents often have "growing pains" that manifest as knee pain. Known clinically as physitis or episphysitis, this condition often targets the knee in particular.

SYMPTOMS

Three basic symptoms can accompany a knee disorder:

- Pain, which is more obvious when walking, especially on stairs; the pain can be stronger going up or going down the stairs.
- Deformity of all or part of the knee joint.
- Inflammation. This will often be due to the effusion of the synovial fluid that lubricates the knee. This condition can appear in any joint but it is of particular importance when it affects the knee.

1. Femur
2. Meniscus
3. Crossed
   ligaments
4. Fibula
5. Patella
6. Synovium
7. Tibia

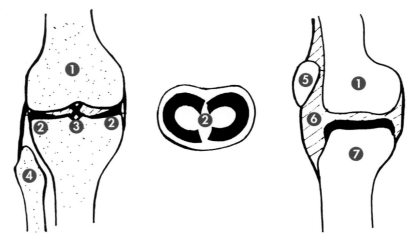

The knee joint

There is one injury that is specific to the knee, the dislocation of one of the two menisces. What this means is that one of the rubbery wedges above the tibia swells up and ruptures. The kick into empty air of a soccer player who misses the ball is the best example of the mechanics of the dislocated meniscus. The most notable sign of a meniscus tear is that the knee locks up when the leg is extended.

Whatever the cause of acute knee pain, an X-ray is almost always necessary for determining the most appropriate therapy.

STANDARD TREATMENT

A variety of treatments exist for the different types of knee problems. Anti-inflammatory medicines and surgeries are among the most common, being necessary for many sprains as well as fractures.

ACUPOINT TREATMENT

There are three specific diagnoses that respond well to acupoint therapy: modest sprains, osteoarthritis pain, and growing pains.

TECHNIQUES TO USE

More than in most other cases, pain in the knee calls for robust stimulation, or an electrical stimulation. Here the therapist has two options: stimulate the points deeply with great force until the pain disappears, or stimulate the points with less intensity for five minutes at a time, two or three times a day. Stimulation can also be applied for several minutes a day as a preventive measure.

The Points

There is one principal point, located three finger-widths above the outside upper edge of the kneecap.

There are three secondary points, two on either side of the bottom tip of the kneecap, and one at the center of the kneecap's top edge.

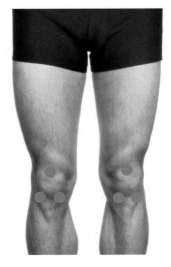
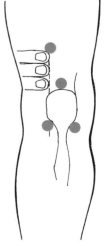

Ankle Disorders

THE ANKLE JOINT consists of four bones: the tibia, the fibula, the talus, and the calcaneous bone. Pathological conditions of the ankle are often traumatic in origin. As the result of a direct shock or more often a forced movement of the foot, something gives—if it is a bone, we are dealing with a fracture, if it involves one or more ligaments then it is a sprain. Radiography often reveals that the two things are combined: a partial fracture accompanied by a sprain, or torn ligaments complicating a broken bone.

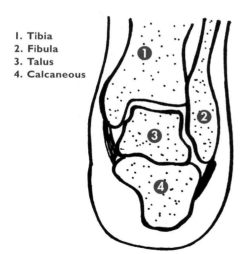

1. Tibia
2. Fibula
3. Talus
4. Calcaneous

Bones of the ankle joint

Fractures and sprains can affect a single bone, only one part of the inner or outer joint, or all of the above. Note that a sprained

ankle should never be neglected. In addition to the pain and initial disability, which may be minor, an ankle that has been injured this way has a tendency to suffer relapses in the future because the ligaments—the mooring posts of the joint—have been torn. From one sprained ankle to the next, we may eventually reach a point where we have an unstable ankle that is constantly swollen and painful—one that will eventually transform the sufferer into a veritable invalid.

STANDARD TREATMENT

While the treatment of fractures is quite standardized, there is no general rule for treating sprains. Some cases will be taped up with ace bandages, or even immobilized in a cast, while other patients will be told to walk at a brisk pace or to soak their feet in alternating baths of hot and cold water. Still others may be advised to ice the injury.

ACUPOINT TREATMENT

Many doctors have been converted into acupuncture fans because of the spectacular speed with which the needles can affect ankle sprains. Whatever other kind of therapy is being applied, acupoint therapy is always worth a try.

TECHNIQUES TO USE

It is appropriate to stimulate the points for ten minutes each hour directly after an injury. Gradually space out the treatments as the swelling in the ankle goes down. With unstable ankles that have suffered repeated sprains, a stimulation of five minutes in the morning and five minutes in the evening should give tone to the ligaments and help prevent relapses.

The Points

There are two principal points, located on the tips of the two ankles.

In addition to these there are two secondary points on both sides of the leg: the first is on the fibula three finger-widths above the outer side of the ankle; the second is on the back edge of the tibia, one hand-width above the inside edge of the ankle, in a small notch.

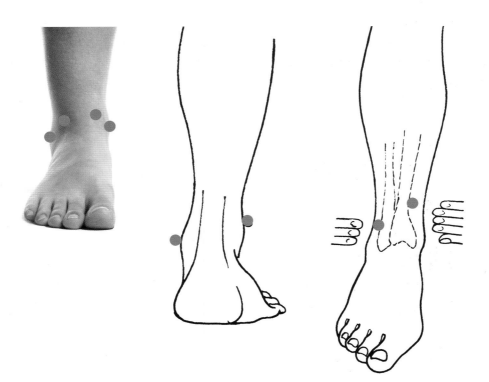

Foot and Toe Disorders

AN EXTRAORDINARY GROUP of twenty-three bones is responsible for bearing the weight of the entire body. Each of these bones in the toes and feet can be affected separately by illness and pain—a sprained or broken toe, for example. But it is quite rare for a part of the foot to be stricken that does not then affect the whole. Why is this? Because this part of the body represents an amazing unit of function. In looking at a foot from the side, and then from the front, note how the burdens it carries are evenly divided between back and front, and between the inside and outside edges. Even the individual structure of each bone reflects this division of labor.

FORMS AND SYMPTOMS

In addition to the common health problems affecting feet and toes like sprains, fractures, and infections, "rheumatism"—in the broad sense of the word—can deform the feet from their regular shape, causing pain and trouble walking. Let's take a look at how these complications appear.

The foot normally rests on a tripod formed by the heel in back and the bottoms of the big and little toes in front. The foot forms an arch between the two front columns. Foot deformities will cause this arch to sink, leaving the weight of the body to rest on the base of all the middle toes, which are not designed to support this load. You can easily imagine the impairment and pain this will cause.

There are two basic deformities that are exact opposites of one another:

The flat foot. Caused by the subsidence of the joints, this causes the entire foot to rest flat upon the ground.
The claw foot (pes cavus). In contrast to the flat foot, this condition occurs when the arch of the foot does not flatten out when bearing weight, and the body rests on the two ends of the foot like a rooster on his spurs.

Deformities may be temporary at first, then become established and have repercussions on the toes. These may deviate radically

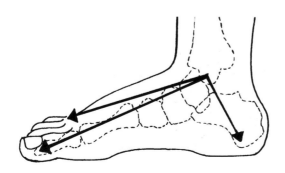

The division of labor: "the tripod."

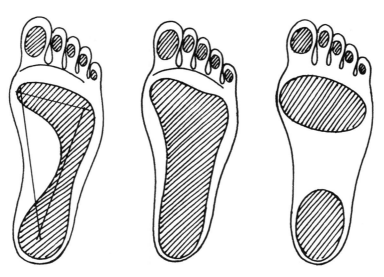

The supports of the foot: normal, with the three points that bear the brunt of the body's weight (left); flat foot (center); claw foot (right)

from their normal condition, with the big toe literally turning inward toward the little toe or outward, and the little toe can do the same. Meanwhile, the other toes will retract, curling in and forming claws. This will cause extreme discomfort, because shoes and the toes themselves will rub against the foot causing corns, calluses, and bunions, which are themselves acutely painful.

CAUSES

This kind of functional disaster can be initially caused by a congenital predisposition. If the muscles of the foot are either too lax or too taut, they will deform the foot's structure early on. This underscores the importance of walking barefoot as often as possible to stabilize muscle tone.

But equal emphasis also has to be put on the deformities that are caused by bad shoes—particularly women's shoes. The

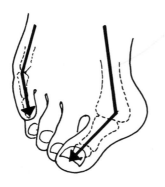
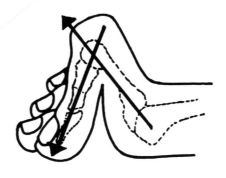

Toe deformities

worst of these are high heels with thin spikes and pointed tips. Oh, ladies, you will only know the true cost of what you are sacrificing for elegance when the deformities are fully established years from now.

STANDARD TREATMENT

In addition to the sedatives that are routinely prescribed in such cases, the foot has to be reeducated to assume its proper position and shape. To do this requires exercising all its joints morning and evening. It is also helpful to support and rebuild a normal arch with soles that raise the heel and cause the bulk of the weight to fall immediately behind the bones that have been displaced.

ACUPOINT TREATMENT

Point stimulation plays both a healing role by fighting pain and a preventive role by keeping the anatomical impairments from becoming established permanently. Because stimulation of the points stimulates the muscles and the ligaments, it restores tone and helps them relax.

TECHNIQUES TO USE

Stimulate these points for a long period of time, perhaps ten or fifteen minutes. Often a simple massage will be enough in the evening when you take off your shoes. This will allow the muscles to relax and the bones to stay in their proper places. An active manipulation of all the joints can be added to finger pressure massage. Pull on your toes, and bend the joints until you hear a cracking sound while you are stimulating the points. This will make the manipulations practically painless. You will be amazed by the results you can see after just a few days of this treatment.

The Principal Point

The principal point is located at the direct center of the top of the foot, halfway between either side.

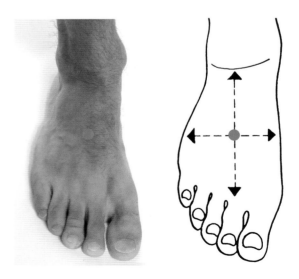

The Secondary Points

The first of the secondary points are located on both sides of the upper edge of the calcaneum bone, between the ankle and the Achilles tendon. These points are quite helpful for treating pain in the heels.

The other points are in the four spaces between the toes, just behind the spot where the toes begin.

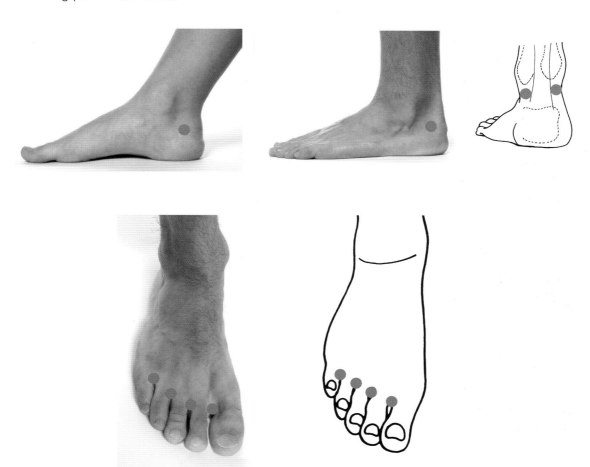

PART FOUR

Digestion

Indigestion and Vomiting

WHO HASN'T VOMITED at some point during their life? Though it's common, and generally merely a passing incident, vomiting can sometimes be a sign of serious illness. Symptoms of vomiting that may need medical attention include large volumes of vomitus (some diseases like cholera cause vomiting of several quarts of liquid and bring about acute dehydration), or repeated vomiting. This is often seen in nursing infants who spit up a large quantity of milk or formula, to the great despair of their mothers. Lastly, vomit containing red blood, or black digested blood, is a sign of a serious health problem.

CAUSES

Sometimes vomiting is merely a symptom of a more deep-seated health problem. Diseases that can have vomiting as a symptom include:

- Problems of a digestive origin—ulcer, cancer of the esophagus or stomach, appendicitis, cholecystitis (inflammation of the gallbladder), liver or pancreas disease.
- Problems of overall health—infections, poisoning, urea, diabetes.
- Problems of nervous origin in the broad sense. Repeated vomiting could be a sign

of meningitis, or of a psychological disease like anorexia, the odd condition that affects young women desperate to remain thin—no matter what the cost.

But fortunately, the vast majority of cases have nothing to do with these grim possibilities and are simply a sign of indigestion, following on the heels of a lavish feast or a night of overdrinking. This indigestion sometimes includes vomiting and even fever.

This brings us to the liver crisis, which is a disease that is specifically French if not uniquely so. What goes under this name is frequently a migraine, an illness that is most frequently hereditary or allergenic. It is the head that causes the liver to feel poorly and not the other way round.

STANDARD TREATMENT

Outside of treating the underlying causes, whenever that is possible, there are now powerful medications that act on the vomiting symptom itself. (These medications can be sleep-inducing, however, which may have its disadvantages—especially for nursing infants.) In addition to treating the symptom, however, it is also necessary to correct the dietary mistakes that led to the problem in the first place. Most cases of indigestion can be brought under control with careful eating for a twenty-four to forty-eight hour period.

ACUPOINT TREATMENT

Acupoint therapy is a wonderfully effective tool for treating vomiting from all causes. For serious vomiting, it can reduce the incidence of vomiting, and thereby reduce the body's fluid loss; it can abbreviate the length and violence of symptoms of indigestion; and it can do a great favor for mothers, who can improve their baby's condition without the help of any drugs.

TECHNIQUES TO USE

For adult indigestion, the first two points have a potent effect. Massage them slowly and with gradually increasing force, pushing on them more and more forcefully, until all the vomiting and reflex vomiting efforts (when there is nothing left to throw up) have disappeared. The last points—those on the fingers—are extremely useful for babies. Once she has finished nursing, the mother should massage them with her fingers. The baby will burp and no longer regurgitate the milk.

The Points

The first point is located on the stomach, halfway between the navel and the lower end of the sternum.

The second point is on the lower part of the leg on the side facing outward, about a hand-width above the ankle. Place your hand over this surface and your thumb will indicate the correct point.

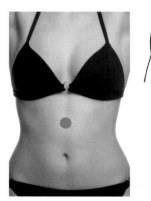
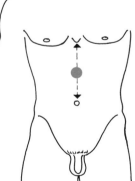
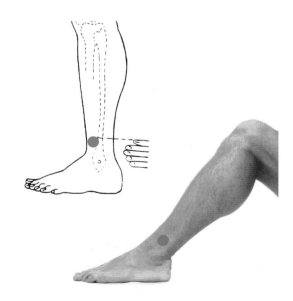

The Points (continued)

The third point—or points, actually, as there are eight of them—are rather unexpected. These points are located on the palm side of the fingers, halfway between the first and second creases of the four fingers of each hand (index, middle, ring, and little finger).

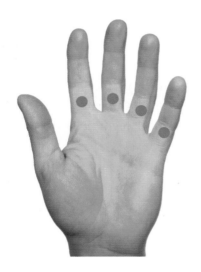
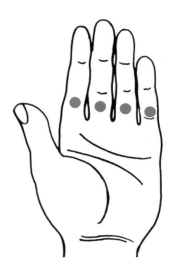

Gallbladder Disorders

THE GALLBLADDER, WHICH is a small pouch hanging beneath the liver, plays the same role in the diet as a dam plays in the irrigation of crops. Because although the liver manufactures bile continuously, it is only needed at the time of digestion, so it must be stored in an organ reservoir that will hold it when it's not useful and release it when needed.

This small organ, the gallbladder—which our ancestors knew as the pouch of venom—is connected to the liver and the intestines by a complex series of canals. The pathology of these canals is almost identical to that of the gallbladder itself, hence we can study both at the same time.

SYMPTOMS

The illnesses connected with the gallbladder reveal their presence with three symptoms: fever, pain, and digestive distress. Sometimes these symptoms are accompanied by a more fickle symptom: a case of jaundice.

The fever is often quite erratic, with periods of calm alternating with brief flare-ups going as high as 104° Fahrenheit. This fever is sometimes called pseudo-malaria, because it brings to mind this tropical disease that is marked by a succession of shivering, high temperatures, and copious sweating.

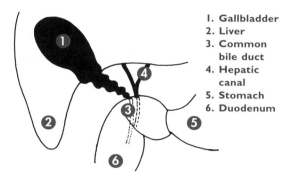

1. Gallbladder
2. Liver
3. Common bile duct
4. Hepatic canal
5. Stomach
6. Duodenum

Gallbladder and surrounding organs

The pain appears in two principal forms, either dull and heavy as if there was a stone beneath the ribs, or, on the contrary, extremely acute, with spasms that cause the sufferer to scream in pain. But in both cases, the pains have one element in common. They travel up the right side of the back and lodge beneath the shoulder blade. This radiation of the pain into the area of the shoulder blade is almost always a sign of its origin in the gallbladder.

The digestive disorders associated with gallbladder disease are quite numerous: diarrhea and/or constipation, nausea and vomiting; quite often aerophagia (air-swallowing) and bloating are also results of a gallbladder disease.

Finally, jaundice can be connected to a gallbladder disorder in a very specific case: when a stone clogs the bile duct.

FORMS AND CAUSES

Gallbladder illnesses can be divided into three categories:

- Acute infections of the gallbladder or bile ducts
- Problems with gallbladder function or biliary dyskinesia
- Bile stones and their complications

Acute inflammation or infection is due to invasion of the gallbladder by intestinal germs. In most cases, a bile stone blocks a duct, which then becomes infected. Fever, acute pain, or vomiting require immediate medical attention and sometimes surgery.

Biliary dyskinesia is a kind of gallbladder disease that occurs without stones. It may be caused by improper contraction of the gallbladder. This organ, like any muscle, needs to contract to empty its contents. These contractions can tend to occur at decreased rates or increased rates, and most often is a combination of the two.

But the biggest problem is bile stones. These stones can occur in any size and in any possible amount. Some are enormous—several grams in size—and occupy the entire interior of the gallbladder, while others are miniscule and seemingly beyond count, forming a kind of biliary mud.

In addition to the functional problems they can cause the gallbladder, these stones can migrate into the bile ducts causing hepatic colic (the painful passage of a bile stone), or block a duct, leading to jaundice or infection as described above.

STANDARD TREATMENTS

Treatments can be divided into those relying on medication and those using surgery.

- Chloecystitis—acute inflammation—often requires massive doses of antibiotics to control the infection, which can otherwise lead to gangrene or peritonitis.
- The problem of biliary dyskinesia has created a huge market for pharmaceutical products called choleretics and cholagogues, gastrointestinal agents that stimulate the flow of bile from the liver and/or gallbladder. In reality, what is called for here is something to synchronize this organ's movement, which medications are ill equipped to do.
- Until recently, gallstones and their complications could only be removed surgically. Some medications have appeared that are able to melt stones inside the gallbladder, but only those that are primarily comprised of cholesterol. These medications have possible side effects making them a risk for certain people.
- Hepatic colic requires the use of the most powerful sedatives, either in the form of pills, suppositories, or shots.

ACUPOINT TREATMENT

Acupoint therapy is most valuable for its ability to synchronize the gallbladder contractions for people suffering from biliary dyskinesia. But it is also capable of treating even the most acutely painful problems like hepatic colic.

TECHNIQUES TO USE

For benign problems, regularly massage the points once in the morning and once in the evening while digesting your meals. Many cases of dyspepsia can disappear this way.

In serious or painful crises (like hepatic colic in particular), stimulate the four points intensely—especially the last one mentioned, using every available technique.

The Principal Points

The first point is located on the outside of the calf, on the front edge of the fibula about a hand-width above the ankle bone; the second is also on the calf, near the knee—a hand-width beneath the crease where you can find a small bone, the head of the fibula. The point is just in front of this area.

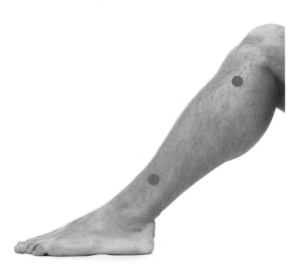

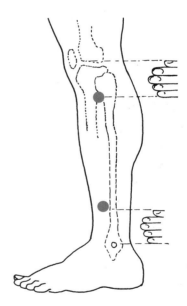

The Secondary Points

The first of the secondary points is located on the back, at the top of the iliac crest, three finger-widths from the spinal column. The point can be found on both sides of the spinal column, but the one on the right side is particularly effective.

The second point is on the leg like the two principal points, but on the inside, one hand-width beneath the crease of the knee in the corner formed by the tibia.

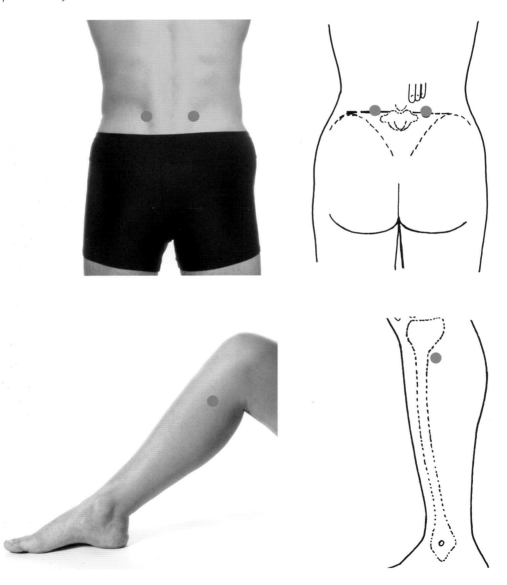

Infectious Hepatitis and Jaundice

HEPATITIS IS AN inflammation of the liver. As a general rule, infectious hepatitis is benign and can be cured leaving no trace in a period of two to three weeks. It is often revealed by, although not synonymous with, jaundice. A yellowish color that appears on the skin and in the eyes, jaundice is due to the deposit of biliary pigment in these parts of the body.

While jaundice is the most obvious symptom of hepatitis, it is by no means the only one; the illness is often accompanied by fever and itching, discoloration of the stools, and a very intense color of the urine: beer brown.

Next, jaundice is not synonymous with infectious hepatitis. There are other diseases capable of causing the same symptoms: some blood anomalies, poisoning, and most importantly the obstruction of the bile ducts, the canals through which bile flows, by a gallstone, for example.

There are also chronic forms of hepatitis. These can gradually eat away the liver and eventually lead to liver cancer or death.

CAUSES

Hepatitis is a viral infection. Intense research has been undertaken on this disease over the last twenty years, and at least five different viruses have been reasonably identified. The three most common viruses are known as hepatitis A, B, and C.

- Hepatitis A is responsible for benign forms of this disease. It can be caught from water and contaminated food.
- Hepatitis B is the cause of the largest number of serious illnesses. It is easily spread by blood transfusions and shared syringes. Today, this contamination frequently has a sexual origin and hepatitis B is today considered to be a venereal disease.
- Hepatitis C is also a cause of many chronic cases of illness. Like hepatitis B, it can be spread via sexual contact or exposure to the blood or body fluids of an infected person.

STANDARD TREATMENT

Many cases of infectious hepatitis resolve by themselves and do not require treatment, but chronic forms of the illness may be treated with antiviral medicines to prevent further damage to the liver.

The best treatment remains prevention: effective vaccines have been developed for hepatitis A and B.

ACUPOINT TREATMENT

Because standard medical treatments are scarce, anything that can provide relief to people suffering from hepatitis is welcome. Acupoint therapy is indeed of this nature and should always be used for hepatitis and jaundice, either with massage or electrical stimulation.

TECHNIQUES TO USE

Stimulate the points for a long period of ten minutes, five to six times a day, until the symptoms improve.

Once the jaundice has gone away, you should still continue stimulating the points for at least a month to eliminate the consequences of hepatitis.

The Principal Points

Both of these points are located on the dorsal spine. The first is beneath the nape of the neck, at the base of the seventh cervical vertebra; the second can be found by tracing a line in between the bottom of the two shoulder blades. The point is along this line on the tip of the spine.

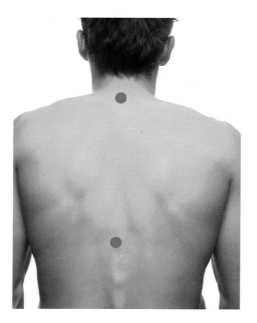
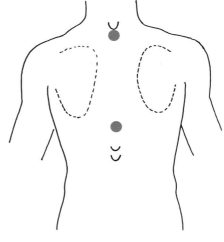

The Secondary Points

The first secondary point is located on the outside aspect of the leg, in front of the head of the small bone that can be felt about a hand-width below the knee; the second point, which can be found on either side of the dorsal spine, is two finger-widths beneath the second principal point.

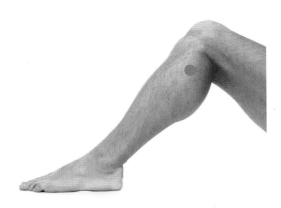

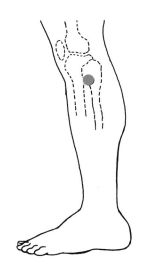

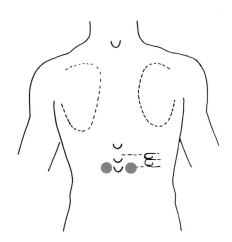

Stomach Pain, Gastritis, and Ulcers

MANY PAINS ORIGINATE in the stomach and the first part of the duodenum, and they can come from many different sources. Attacks on the top part of the small intestine, which is called the duodenum, and the pylorus (the border zone between the stomach and the intestine) cause practically the same symptoms as ailments of the stomach itself, and can be confused for them. It is also important to note that diverse conditions of the abdomen and chest can cause the epigastrium to feel poorly, including diseases of the gallbladder, the liver, the pancreas, even the heart and the pleura.

For this reason it is a good idea to consult a physician to determine the actual cause of any pain that you may be feeling in the epigastric region.

SYMPTOMS

Stomach pain always occurs with the same symptoms: cramps, burning sensations, and heartburn.

Furthermore, it is generally in tune with meal times, and can come on right before eating, when one is fasting, or sometime afterward, when you are digesting your food. Pain can be accompanied by other symptoms

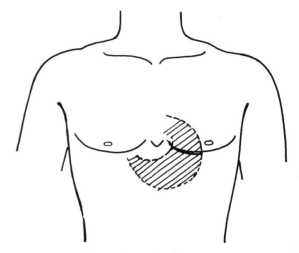

Stomach projection zone

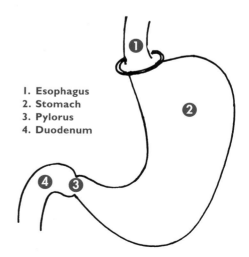

1. Esophagus
2. Stomach
3. Pylorus
4. Duodenum

Anatomy of the stomach area

such as burping, nausea, somewhat acidic vomiting, or even by the appearance of very different symptoms like asthma crises or chest pains.

CAUSES

There are four principal causes for the pain in the epigastric area: ulcers, gastritis, hiatal hernia, and the excruciating stomach cancer. Ulcers are holes in the stomach lining that can be caused either by excessive amounts of acid or *H. pylori* bacteria. Anxiety may also play a role in the development of ulcers (it is commonly said that a person has an ulcer in the head before having one in the stomach). Another now common origin lies in medications like cortisone or anti-inflammatory drugs.

Gastritis is due to inflammation of the mucous membrane, which can be a result of poor stomach function or of attacks on the lining of the stomach by tobacco, alcohol, coffee, hot peppers, and so on.

The origin of hiatal hernias, meanwhile, is a structural problem in the upper part of the stomach cavity. When the diaphragm muscle has poor tone, part of the stomach can penetrate into the chest, which interferes with the stomach's ability to function properly.

STANDARD TREATMENT

Medical treatment in the grand majority of cases relies on antacids, acid blockers, and proton pump inhibitors. Surgery for any

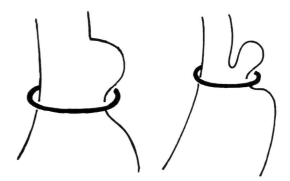

Depiction of paraesophageal hiatal hernia (left) and sliding hiatal hernia (right)

of these conditions has become quite rare, except in cases of stomach cancer, for which it is imperative.

ACUPOINT TREATMENT

Although medications can be quite effective, acupoint therapy has an important role in treating these ailments. It can help patients to avoid recurrences of their symptoms, and even help reduce the need for medications. In most cases, acupoint therapy can be remarkably soothing for digestive troubles including bloating, pain, abdominal noises, and so forth.

TECHNIQUES TO USE

To treat chronic epigastric symptoms, stimulate the points two or three times a day, for fifteen minutes each time. In China, they often use methods of continuous stimulation—like electrical stimulation units—for this kind of ailment.

The Principal Points

The first principal point is located on the palm side of the wrist, right at the center, three finger-widths below the wrist crease; the second is on the outer side of the calf, one hand-width beneath the crease of the knee.

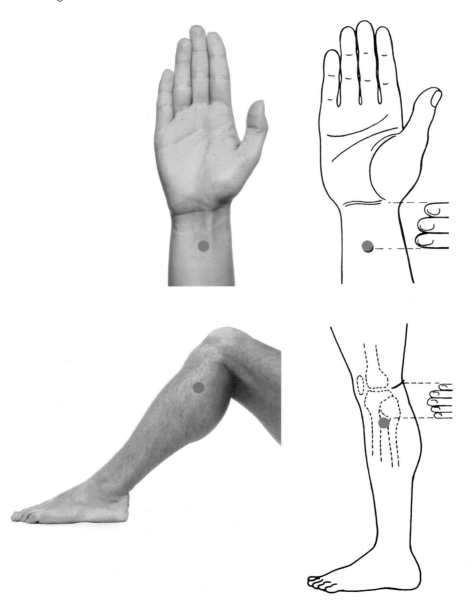

The Secondary Points

The first of the secondary points is located in the middle of the line connecting the navel to the lower end of the sternum. The second point is on the midpoint of the back, two finger-widths away from the center of the spine.

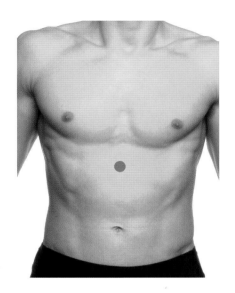

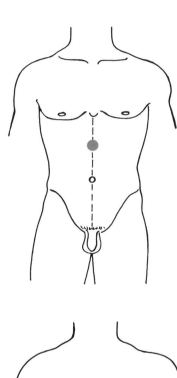

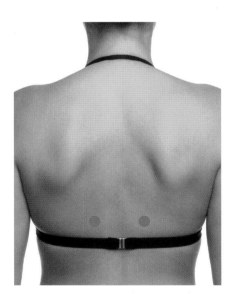

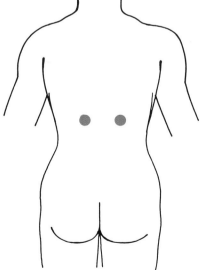

Constipation and Colitis

CONSTIPATION—THE ABSENCE OF a daily bowel movement—is one of the true diseases of modern civilization. As Madame de Recamier said (as quoted by Sainte-Beuve): "They do not all die, but all were wounded . . ." It is very rare for anyone to not have experienced periods of constipation during their life. But constipation also falls into the much larger context of *colitis,* which is the clinical term for inflammation of the large intestine.

We shall see what is truly meant by this far-too-vague term, which is used a bit too freely by modern gastroenterology.

FORMS AND SYMPTOMS

There are two standard forms of constipation: atonic constipation (lazy bowel), in which the individual can go for eight days without defecating and without feeling any discomfort from this, and spastic constipation, which is accompanied by pain, diarrhea, and other symptoms.

In reality, these two forms basically correspond to two different portions of the bowel: atonic constipation is related to the anus whereas spastic constipation is connected to the poor functioning of the large intestine, and is therefore a form of colitis.

Careful study is required when someone is constipated. First of all, how many bowel movements is the person having each day? The appropriate number will vary from one individual to the next. If someone is not "going" every day, is it every two days, three days, or even less often? What are the stools like? Are they small and fragmentary or, to the contrary, quite large? Are there severe diarrhea episodes from time to time? Are there accompanying symptoms like pain and bloating?

Finally, and most importantly, is the constipation new or old? Constipation that has been an enduring feature of an individual's life since childhood—while annoying—is not fundamentally serious, whereas a case of constipation that has recently appeared should prompt one to hunt down its exact cause.

CAUSES

Atonic constipation is a side effect of a deficiency in the anus, which is clinically described as rectal dyschezia. Here is where the illnesses of modern civilization find their chief causes—meals that are irregular in size and eaten at irrregular hours, too many rich foods like meat, sweets, and sauces, insufficient liquids, and inadequate exercise all contribute to dulling the defecation reflex, which the body eventually "forgets." There is also an entire psychological background at play here: anxiety causes the sphincters to clench up. Nervous individuals have a tendency to hold as tight to their stools as they do to everything else. Freud constructed an entire part of his theory on the "anal stage"; breaking through this stage represents one of the major transitional events of individual development.

We also have more prosaic causes of atonic constipation. Can anyone say if the replacement of "Turkish toilets" with English toilets may not have contributed to the creation of more constipation because they caused us to abandon a more physiologically favorable position for defecation?

Spastic constipation is more a side effect of an affliction that targets the large intestine: colitis. However, this term *colitis* has become a catch-all word that conceals a number of various causes. Colitis can be a secondary symptom of:

- A benign or malignant tumor; this is important to bear in mind when suffering from a recent onset of constipation
- Parasites such as protozoa, candida, worms, and so on
- A veritable poisoning of the intestine by antibiotics, which have either been prescribed in excess amounts or taken for too long a time

Generally speaking, however, colitis is a disease of nervous origin. Conditions of spastic colitis or irritable bowel serve as a kind of "mirror to the soul." The contractions alternate with a decrease in gastrointestinal transit time, which explains the constipation.

Constipation and colitis are often present over an entire lifetime, with phases of improvement alternating with aggravated periods connected to the normal incidents of life. But we need to be aware that there is more to the problem of constipation than the discomfort of not feeling suitably "emptied." Constipation is increasingly viewed as a chief culprit responsible for two of the main scourges of the modern world—cancers, especially those of the intestine, because of the chronic irritation caused by the presence of stagnant stools; and high cholesterol, because the overdigestion of matter in the intestines frees up a greater quantity of cholesterol.

STANDARD TREATMENT

First, here is what you should not do: *do not take laxatives.* These products are the basis for one of the most widespread health problems in the world today: laxative abuse, which robs the body of water and minerals and can be fatal in the worst cases.

Instead, what is necessary is a change of lifestyle and a change of diet, incorporating food with a lot of roughage, like green vegetables. Fiber is particularly good for constipation, and its recent re-entry into the popular lexicon represents a huge step forward therapeutically.

ACUPOINT TREATMENT

For health problems that are this insidious and chronic, it is of enormous value to have within hand's reach a simple and effective method like acupoint therapy. I have no hesitation in saying that it should be the first treatment option to be chosen. By way of example, I would like to quickly mention the story of one of my own patients, a twelve-year-old boy who was stricken with rectal paralysis. He was given a regular massage that stimulated the appropriate pressure points, which permitted him to have a daily bowel movement.

TECHNIQUES TO USE

Start establishing a regular time for bowel movements and at that time, strongly massage the principal points described below. In order to reeducate the intestine, it is best to stimulate the different points one after the other for two minutes each, once in the morning and once in the evening.

The second point is particularly effective for treating painful episodes of colitis and should be stimulated three times a day.

The Principal Points

The first of these points is located on the side of the big toe facing the other toes, at the corner of the nail; the second point is on the out-ward facing side of the leg, about a hand-width beneath the crease of the knee, below and in front of the small head of the fibula bone.

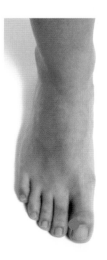
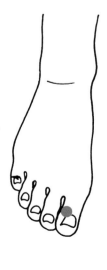
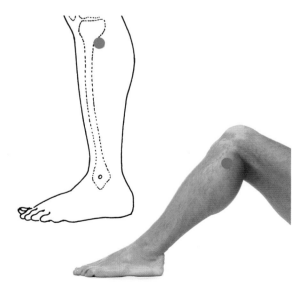

The Secondary Points

The first secondary point is on the stomach, level with the navel and four finger-widths to either side of it. The second point is on the inner side of the leg beneath the knee, in the corner of the tibia bone.

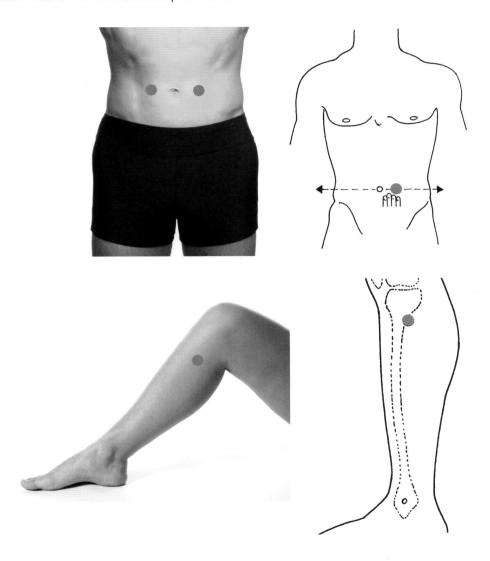

Diarrhea

DIARRHEA IS THE evacuation of liquid stools. The stools can vary in consistency from completely liquid to a pasty puree, or they can be a mixture of liquid and more solid fragments. The color of such stools can be brown, yellow, or green, and they can contain varying degrees of blood, phlegm, and fat. It is important to note that episodic acute diarrhea following an attack of indigestion has nothing in common with chronic diarrhea, in which the stools are abnormal day after day after day.

CAUSES

Acute attacks of diarrhea are almost always connected to an outside cause: food intolerance or a bacterial or microbial infection. Some of these infections can be quite serious, such as bacillary dysentery (shigellosis) or amoebic dysentery (amoebiasis).

Chronic diarrhea is more often connected with health problems affecting the pancreas, the small intestine, or the large intestine. I would like to emphasize two forms of chronic diarrhea in particular:

- The first is due to two diseases of unknown origin, whose presence is revealed by bloody stools: ulcerative colitis and Crohn's Disease.

- The second is connected with the bad habit of taking laxatives on a regular basis; these pharmaceutical substances trigger the release of liquid stools that empty the individual's body of its water and mineral salts. This is a very unhealthy habit, impossible to advise against too strongly.

STANDARD TREATMENT

The standard treatment for diarrhea varies, of course, depending on what caused it. Medications to fight infection or parasites are prescribed when it is due to an outside cause, but when the cause is internal, physicians strive to restore regular organ function. In serious cases, rehydration by IV needs to be performed at a hospital.

ACUPOINT TREATMENT

While acupoint therapy makes no claims of treating the very causes of diarrhea, it does play a useful role in reducing the loss of fluids and raising intestinal function to a more appropriate level.

TECHNIQUES TO USE

Vigorous repeated massages are the best approach to treating acute diarrhea. These should be done several minutes every hour and often will halt the evacuation of liquid stools.

On the other hand, chronic diarrhea calls for even more continuous stimulation. Try fifteen minutes of massage, three to four times per day.

The Principal Points

The first point is on the edge of the index finger facing the thumb, above the first finger joint; the second is located on the outer side of the calf, ten centimeters below the knee crease. We may also find this point at the junction of the upper third and the two lower thirds of the leg.

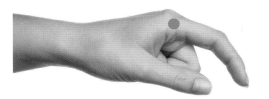

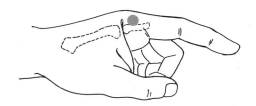

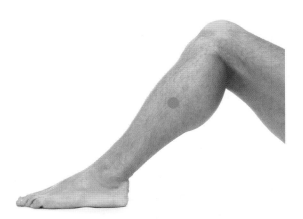

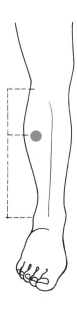

The Secondary Points

The first of the secondary points is at the outer end of the elbow crease. The other point is on the stomach, two finger-widths below the navel.

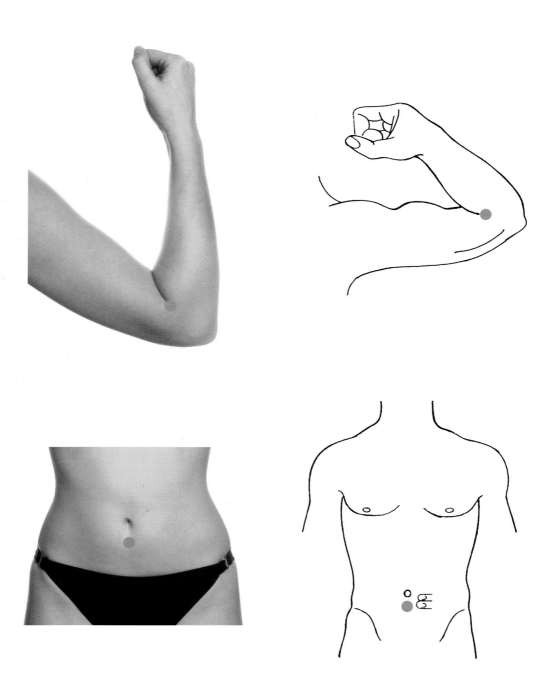

Hemorrhoids and
Other Problems of the Anus

HEMORRHOIDS ARE THE most common health problem affecting the anus. They are basically a form of varicose vein, appearing on the anus. Veins are a normal feature of the anus and circle it completely: these veins are known as the hemorrhoidal veins. When these veins dilate they become hemorrhoids.

SYMPTOMS AND FORMS

The three essential signs of hemorrhoids are pain, bleeding, and oozing. The pain is generally a dull, heavy pain that increases during bowel movements. This is the time the hemorrhoids bleed, accompanying the fecal matter with a jet of bright red blood. Between bowel movements, the anus remains moist because of the oozing, which is often irritating and can smell bad. These are simple hemorrhoids, but complications can arise that make matters worse.

Sometimes a small clot forms that creates a hemorrhoidal thrombosis, a little painful ball that can appear either inside or outside the anus. The hemorrhoids can become inflamed, in which case it is a hemorrhoidal anitis. Sometimes, they "emerge" out of the anus as a compact mass creating a hemorrhoidal prolapse.

But hemorrhoids are not the only disorders that can affect the anus. In addition to annoying symptoms like anal itching, I would like to draw your attention to two other potentially serious conditions: anal fissures and anal fistulas.

An anal fissure is a painful crack or tear in the skin of the anal canal. An anal fistula is a small oozing orifice located within close proximity of the anus; it may discharge a kind of pus. Fistulas can be the cause of extremely serious abscesses.

Itching in the anal region can be the consequence of earlier diseases, but it can also

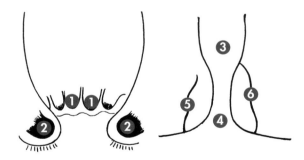

1. Hemorrhoidal veins
2. Anal sphincter muscles
3. Rectum
4. Anal canal
5. Blind fistula (has only one open end and does not connect with the intestine)
6. Complete fistula (provides a channel from the skin to intestine)

Cross section of the anus

appear independently. If a child complains of anal itching, he or she should be evaluated for intestinal worms. In adults, anal itching can be a sign of a fungal infection, or diabetes. Finally, you should be especially wary of any abnormal manifestation in this region of the body that could be a sign of tumors. Know when to consult a specialist (in this case it would be the proctologist), especially when these major warning signs appear: hemorrhages of black blood that appear between bowel movements.

CAUSES

Constipation was long considered the chief cause of hemorrhoids, thought to exert undue force upon the veins, making them varicose. In reality, it would seem that diarrhea is more often to blame. Let's just say that all digestive disorders can trigger an outbreak, as well as anything that obstructs the blood in the veins (pregnancy for example).

Anal fissures and fistulas, meanwhile have a very different origin. Fissures are generally the result of a tear in the mucous membrane; this is most often caused by pushing too hard to evacuate the stool. Fistulas are attributed to a birth defect that has allowed small "pouches" to form that open to the skin and sometimes the intestine.

STANDARD TREATMENT

An outbreak of hemorrhoids is generally treated by phlebotonic medications, which is to say medications that restore tone to the veins, combined with anti-inflammatory preparations. These medications can be taken orally or applied locally either as an ointment or a suppository.

A thrombotic hemorrhoid (also known as piles) requires immediate removal and is usually incised like a small abscess. Laser surgery is often an option here. Removal of this small painful "ball" will provide immediate relief.

When hemorrhoid outbreaks start occurring too frequently or the hemorrhoids are too large, doctors often prescribe a radical treatment called sclerosis, which involves injecting the hemorrhoids with substances that will cause them to thicken and harden, and make it easier for them to be surgically extracted.

Anal fissures and fistulas have specific treatments: shots of relaxants in the first case, traction with stitches for the second. Pruritus (itching), however, is often a source of despair for its sufferers and their doctors. Few effective treatments are available.

ACUPOINT TREATMENT

Acupoint therapy can often effectively relieve an acute case of hemorrhoids; it also provides greater relief during an anal fissure crisis. Finally, used regularly, acupoint therapy often has a powerful effect on alleviating pruritus, and can lengthen the interval between hemorrhoid outbreaks.

TECHNIQUES TO USE

Massage or stimulate the principal points vigorously when an acute case of hemorrhoids occurs, until you feel complete relief.

If necessary, repeat the stimulation after several minutes.

For chronic problems, including itching, the stimulation should be repeated two or three times a day, in five- to ten-minute sessions.

The Principal Points

The first point is located midway up the calf, in the center of the muscle mass. The second principal point is at the tip of the coccyx.

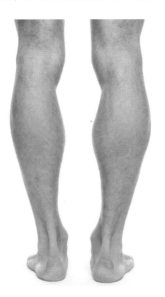 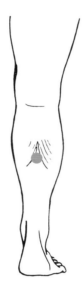 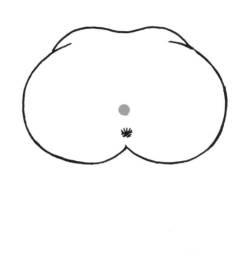

The Secondary Points

The first of these points is located on the upper lip below the nose; the second is at the very top of the head (at the tallest point of the body), at the junction of the median line and the line passing over the top of the auricles of both ears. It should be noted that this point has remarkable effectiveness in treating hemorrhoidal prolapse.

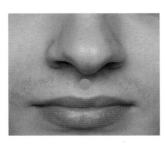 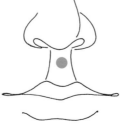 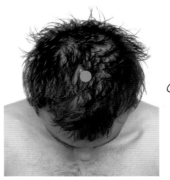 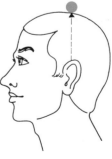

PART FIVE

Circulation

High Blood Pressure

THE CURRENT DEFINITION for adult high blood pressure, or hypertension, is when the arterial pressure, read with the standard cuff monitor, is 140/90 or higher. Normal blood pressure is considered to be 120/80, so anything within this range is considered pre-hypertension—an indication that the patient is at risk. The final figure should be based on three successive readings.

Sometimes the person suffering from hypertension will be alerted to its existence by headaches, problems with eyesight, and so on. But as a general rule, high blood pressure is "mute" and only discovered by a doctor during the course of a routine examination. For this reason, it is important that three or four readings be taken before it is confirmed.

CAUSES

Some high blood pressure cases are due to a precise cause, such as a tumor in the adrenal glands or serious kidney disease, but these are the exceptions.

The majority of "essential" hypertension cases—meaning those with no obvious cause—are actually caused by extremely complex disorders of certain hormones or related substances found in the blood. The role of these chemicals (renin, aldosterone, angiotensin) is very complicated and still being studied. In addition, an individual's psychological state can be a factor in hypertension.

STANDARD TREATMENT

When treatment is called for, different kinds of pharmaceutical medications are used:

- Some act to "empty" the body of water and salt; these are diuretics.
- Others prevent blood pressure from rising; these are called beta-blockers.
- Others, finally, act on the hormones implicated in hypertension, which we discussed above, by inhibiting their activity.

Whatever course of action is chosen, it is the opinion of standard medicine that the patient will require this treatment for the duration of his or her life. This is difficult to enforce because the patient does not feel sick and may not feel drugs are necessary, especially as they may have all kinds of disadvantageous side effects, the most notable of which is sexual impotence.

ACUPOINT TREATMENT

Acupoint therapy has little effect on the complex cases of hypertension involving cardiac and renal disorders, but it can be fully effective in mild and temporary cases of high blood pressure. Even in moderate cases, it offers a valuable complementary treatment that can help reduce the amount of medication a patient needs.

TECHNIQUES TO USE

As this is a chronic ailment, it is appropriate to stimulate the points for several minutes (five to seven minutes), two or three times a day. More continuous stimulation via electrical current is even more effective and has revolutionized high blood pressure treatment.

The Principal Points

The first is located on the back edge of the skull, inside a small notch about two finger-widths behind the ear. The second point is on the outer end of the elbow crease.

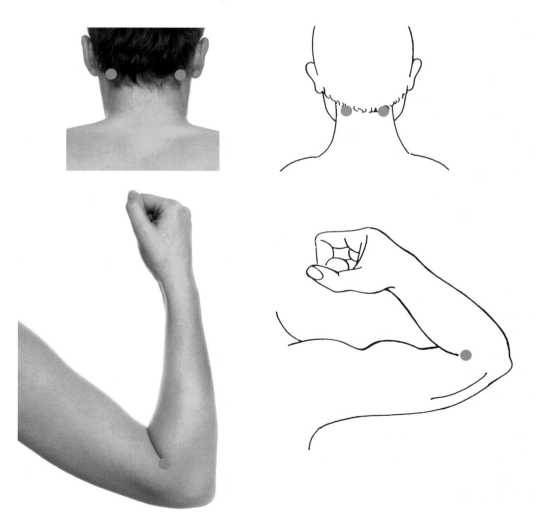

The Secondary Points

The first secondary point is in the notch formed where the bones leading into the big toe and the second toe meet on the foot. The second point is on the outside of the calf, one hand-width beneath the crease of the knee.

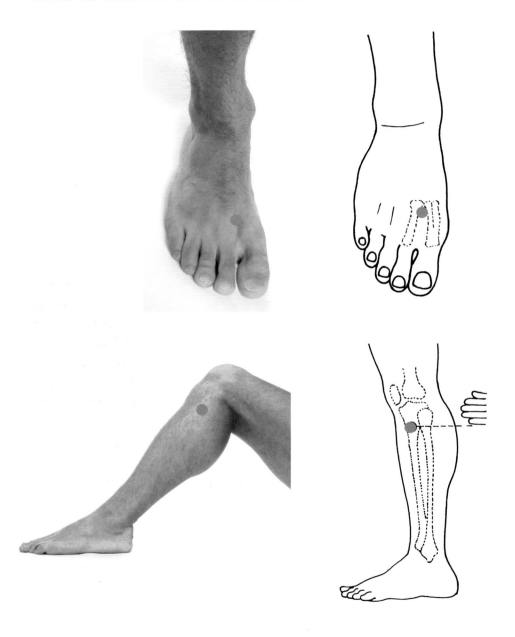

Heart Failure

WHEN THE HEART muscle is no longer capable of effectively performing its task as a pump moving blood throughout the body, the other organs will suffer from deficiencies of oxygen. Although the heart keeps pumping, it does not do so with adequate force or frequency. As a general rule, this stage is, in fact, the terminal development of many heart and lung diseases.

A certain number of symptoms provide almost constant indications of heart failure. These occur in parts of the body that serve as reservoirs when the blood forms deposits. They include:

- The legs, which become swollen with edema.
- The liver, which increases in size and often causes digestive disorders. When it reaches a certain terminal state it has been described as resembling an accordion.
- The lungs, which can become suddenly flooded with blood and require emergency treatment, or they can become gradually engorged with fluid, creating respiratory distress that can be mistaken for bronchitis.

In sum, the trinity here is edema, enlarged liver, and dyspnea (respiratory distress). There are also other signs that reveal the exhaustion of the heart muscle itself:

- The heart starts racing to compensate with speed for what its power can no longer do: this is tachycardia.
- The heart grows larger: this is especially visible in X-rays.

FORMS AND CAUSES

It is standard to make a distinction between right-sided heart failure, which impairs the ability of the heart to send blood to the lungs, and left-sided heart failure, in which the rest of the organ is failing. In fact, it is most often the entire heart that is failing.

As I noted earlier, heart failure is the terminal phase in the development of a number of lung and heart diseases. I will mention the lung diseases first as the lung is a veritable sponge for blood. When the passage of blood through this organ meets resistance, it causes the heart to overwork and eventually exhaust itself. This leads to right-sided then overall heart failure. This is what happens with chronic bronchitis and emphysema, and other conditions affecting the lungs.

Next are the diseases that affect the heart directly. Among these, the most frequent are those affecting the heart valves, heart attacks, and certain illnesses affecting the heart muscle itself (myocardiopathies).

STANDARD TREATMENT

Standard medical treatments tend to focus on two objectives: first, to reduce body fluids as much as possible in order to ease the strain on the "pump." Hence a salt-free diet and diuretics, which reduce edema by causing urination. Second, medications like digitalis and nitrites are used to restore the tone of the heart muscle.

ACUPOINT TREATMENT

Let me say straight off that the role of acupoint therapy is quite modest here; it can only be a complement to other therapies. However, it is never dangerous and always useful, as it makes it possible to lower the intake of certain chemical medications.

TECHNIQUES TO USE

As this is a chronic illness, it is necessary to stimulate the points in a constant if not permanent manner, or if this is not possible, to repeat the stimulation several times a day (three times on average) for four or five minutes at a time.

The Principal Point

The principal point is located on the palm's "heart line," at the point where it can be touched by the tip of the little finger.

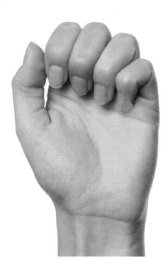

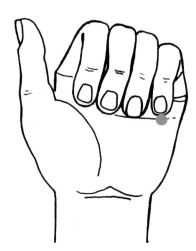

The Secondary Points

The first is located on the palm side of the wrist, three finger-widths beneath the crease; the second is on the back, two finger-widths on either side of the tip of the fourth thoracic vertebra. To locate this vertebra, count down four vertebrae from the seventh cervical vertebra, whose location is described in detail at the end of the introduction. (See page 9.)

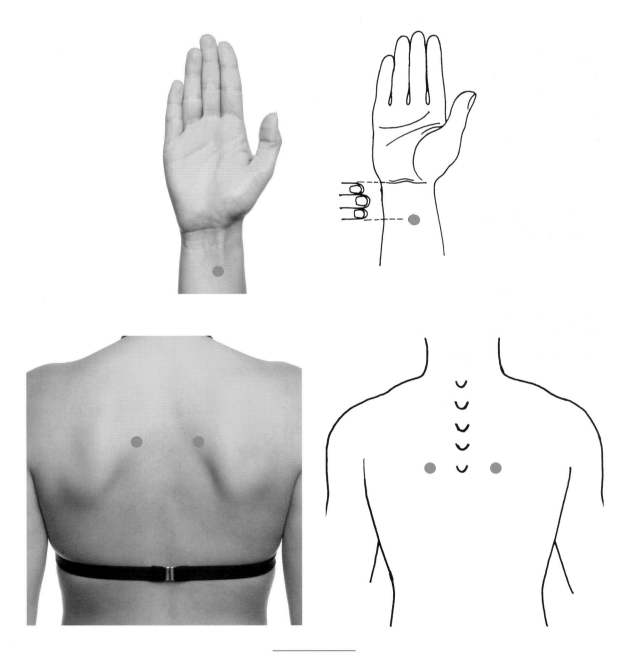

Peripheral Vascular Disease

PERIPHERAL VASCULAR DISEASE refers to the hardening of arteries other than the heart. The term is widely used to describe conditions of the leg arteries in particular. As a result of reduced circulation, the muscles and skin of the legs are no longer irrigated with blood, which can have serious consequences.

SYMPTOMS

The first sign of peripheral vascular disease—and often it is the only sign for a long time—is pain. But this is a very distinctive kind of pain as it may only be felt during walking. The sufferer can walk for four hundred or six hundred feet, when she will suddenly feel a painful cramp in her calves that forces her to stop. After a brief rest, the cramps go away, and the individual can resume walking, only to be forced to a halt again after walking another four hundred feet. This phenomenon is known as "intermittent claudication." Another odd and unusual symptom is that the feet grow colder at the same time, which is the opposite of what normally happens when walking. The more the patient walks, the colder the feet become, until they are completely numb.

CAUSES

Peripheral vascular disease is a manifestation of arteriosclerosis. This illness can often be traced back to two main causes: diabetes and tobacco. If either of these is indeed the cause, the first should be treated and the second eliminated.

STANDARD TREATMENT

Fortunately, modern medical treatments now make it possible to avoid the worst consequences of this disease in the vast majority of cases. In addition to eliminating tobacco and addressing diabetes, if it is a factor, standard medical treatment consists of pharmaceutical products for dilating the arteries or thinning the blood. If these methods do not work, the next option is surgery. Here surgeons generally create a bypass, circumventing the obstructed zone by using a kind of plastic hose. In favorable cases, a catheter equipped with a small balloon is inserted in the artery then inflated at the stricken area to remove the obstruction. These operations perform veritable miracles, but they are always major surgical interventions and the patient must be monitored carefully the rest of her life. And unfortunately, the arteries so treated will often clog again.

ACUPOINT TREATMENT

Acupoint therapy has an important role to play here because it can prompt a controlled dilation of the arteries. Of course, it cannot open an artery that is completely blocked, but it can improve the remaining network enough to assure the leg a sufficient supply of blood. For this reason it should be systematically combined with the standard treatments. It is a good idea to monitor the improvement in a patient's condition, for example by noting the increasing distance one can walk, and by repeating the common Doppler test.

TECHNIQUES TO USE

As this is a chronic affliction, frequent stimulations are required for several minutes at a time, two or three times a day. A more continuous form of stimulation, such as electrical stimulation, is also an option here.

The Principal Points

The first point is located on a place that can be quite hard to reach: immediately behind the anus. The second is in the notch formed where the bones leading into the big toe and the second toe meet on the foot.

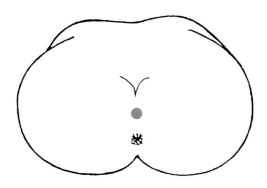
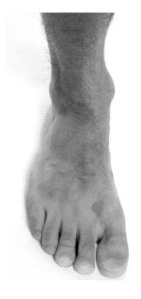
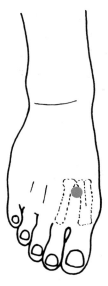

The Principal Points (continued)

The third point is on the top of the thigh. With the leg bent, place your palm on the kneecap and rest your fingers on the thigh. Your index finger will indicate the correct point.

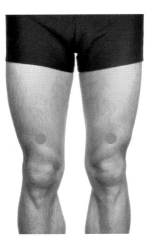
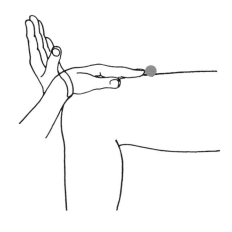

The Secondary Points

The secondary points are located at the base of the toes, in the spaces that separate them.

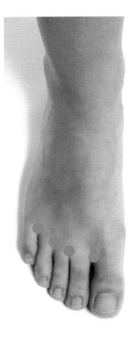
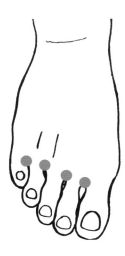

Venous Insufficiency: Varicose Veins, Swollen Legs, Thromboses

IT IS COMMON knowledge that the heart sends blood into the tissues via the arteries, then nourishes them by virtue of the capillaries before the blood returns to the heart by means of the veins. Any problems with the return circulation are therefore essentially disorders of the veins.

There are two types of vein circulation through the lower limbs. One is deeply buried within the muscles, practically next to the bone, while the other is a superficial course that winds its way beneath the skin.

The major health problem that can happen in this area is the obstruction of a vein corked by a blood clot. When this happens, it is a thrombosis—a deep vein thrombosis if it attacks the deep vein sector, and a superficial vein thrombosis if it affects the superficial network beneath the skin. In addition to this acute disorder, we can also have problems caused by passive vein dilation, better known as varicose veins.

All kinds of complications are possible from these health disorders: swollen legs, heavy legs, varicose ulcers, and so forth. We shall now take a closer look at each of these disorders.

SYMPTOMS AND FORMS

Deep vein thrombosis most often occurs following surgery or giving birth, or as a result of long distance travel by car or plane, or lengthy bed rest. A person may have no symptoms, or may experience redness, warmth, swelling, or pain in all or part of the leg. The biggest risk associated with deep vein thrombosis is the possibility of part of the clot breaking off and traveling to the lungs, where it can trigger a pulmonary embolism.

Superficial vein thrombosis is an entirely different story. As the result of a blow or injury to the foot, and sometimes even spontaneously, a red patch appears on the calf, which should not be mistaken for an abscess. This quickly forms into a kind of cord in which the vein becomes harder and transforms into a hard, red, and painful string. The blood clot is beneath the skin in the upper part of this cord.

The initial appearance of varicose veins is described as varicosity—a fine threadlike network appearing in different spots on the legs and thighs. Then a vein, which until this time had been barely visible beneath the skin, swells up until it can actually resemble a snake winding its way down the thigh and leg.

A full range of sensations starting with "heavy legs," then swelling and edema precedes this phase. These symptoms first come on at night, then progress to permanent status. They are often, unfortunately, accompanied by a large number of complications including ochre pigmentation of the leg, swelling that can result in the formation of a veritable boot of skin clamped around the leg, and most particularly varicose ulcers— small holes that are generally located around the ankles, which can be excruciatingly painful and extremely hard to get rid of.

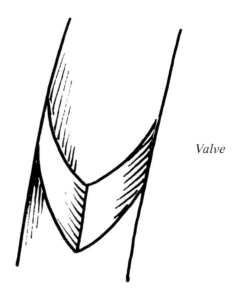

Valve

CAUSES

Deep vein thrombosis is connected with a blood coagulation problem, which creates an obstructing clot.

The mechanism of varicose veins is more complex. In order to really grasp it, you need to keep in mind the circulatory return system and the structure of the veins. The blood in the veins, in contrast to that in the arteries, is under no pressure. Its return to the heart can only be achieved by movements of the limb, which are then transmitted to the vein. As a consequence, blood can just as easily fall back into the feet as it can continue its progression toward the heart. To prevent this ebb, small valves exist in the veins to force the blood to flow toward the heart. When these valves are impaired or overworked, the veins become varicose and set the stage for further complications like swollen legs and ulcers.

STANDARD TREATMENT

Anticoagulant treatments have had a stunning effect in reversing the development of thromboses, and are even used as a preventive measure during and after surgery. This treatment is not necessary for superficial vein thromboses, however; those require anti-inflammatory medications and, if necessary, the surgical extraction of the small blood clot.

The treatment of varicose veins is more complex. Compression stockings or injection of the veins with a sclerosing solution that causes them to wither away are two alternatives to having them removed surgically. The veins may require the sclerosing treatment on a constant basis, once a year on average, because the varicose veins keep reforming. Sclerotherapy and surgery are often performed in tandem as they are complementary.

ACUPOINT TREATMENT

Acupoint therapy does not have a vital role to play in the treatment of deep or superficial thromboses, but it can serve as a kind of backup.

When it comes to varicose veins, the picture is a little more hopeful. While point stimulation has little effect on the varicose dilations themselves, it is quite effective at lessening the symptoms associated with them including the sensation of heavy legs, swellings or edemas, and even varicose ulcers. Its regular use brings about substantial improvement in these symptoms and can even help prevent them from appearing.

TECHNIQUES TO USE

Stimulation with finger massage should be given repeatedly, for ten minutes three times a day, and even longer if the leg is swollen. Ongoing stimulation with an electrical device is worth trying, especially at night.

The Principal Points

The first point is located on the top of the foot, in the notch formed by the two bones leading to the big toe and its neighbor.

The second point is on the top of the thigh. With the leg bent, place your palm on the kneecap, then fold your fingers around the knee. Your index finger will indicate the correct point.

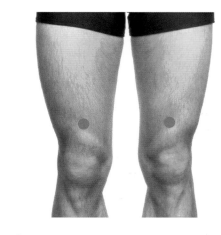

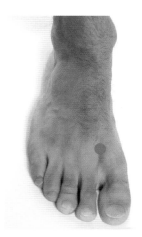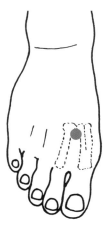

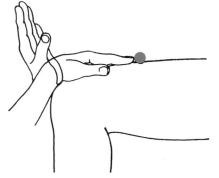

The Secondary Points

The first secondary point is located on the crease at the top of the foot, against the inner edge of the ankle; the second is on the top of the wrist crease, on the palm and thumb side.

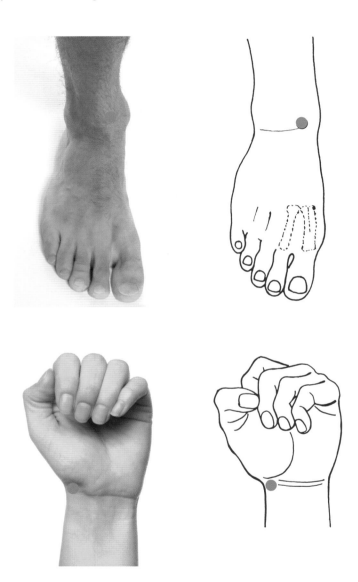

PART SIX

Urinary System

Nephritic Colic
and Kidney Stones

NEPHRITIC COLIC IS an intense pain that generally comes on quite violently along the length of the right or left urinary tract, as a rule caused by the movement of a kidney stone. In the vast majority of cases, the pain appears quite suddenly or within a period of several minutes.

It is intense and terrible and always follows the same course. The pain starts from one of the kidneys (which are located higher than is commonly believed, beneath the ribs), travels down through the lumbar region and

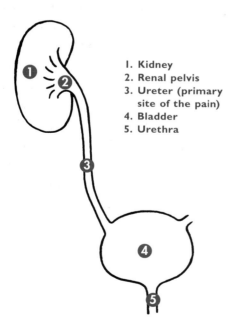

1. **Kidney**
2. **Renal pelvis**
3. **Ureter (primary site of the pain)**
4. **Bladder**
5. **Urethra**

The path of pain in nephritic colic

the stomach to end in the genital region—in other words along the course of the ureter that carries urine from the kidney into the bladder.

The sufferer often writhes in agony while futilely trying to find a position that will relieve the pain—but nothing brings relief. A number of additional problems can add to the individual's misery. There are digestive complications (vomiting, gas, diarrhea, and so forth) as well as urinary problems. The sufferer has repeated desires to urinate but can only squeeze out a few drops, which are often bloody.

Despite the violence of the pain, it is far better to have a full-blown crisis that pushes the stone along the ureter than the less severe episodes in which the ureter and then the upper urinary tracts can become distended, thus endangering the kidney itself.

CAUSES

As we saw above, the vast majority of the cases of nephritic colic are due to the passage of a kidney stone down through the ureter.

Stones are formed in the renal pelvis for a variety of reasons, not all of which have yet been determined. Generally, high levels of mineral salts in the urine are thought to contribute to the formation of stones, the way hard water will cake the plumbing with lime scaling. Kidney stones start off as quite small and first appear as "sand" or "urinary sludge." These little crystals then combine together and eventually form real pebbles of varied form and size.

The chemical nature of these stones also varies. Depending on the individual case, the individual may be dealing with a uric, calcic, oxalic, cystinic, or magnesium stone. This has an important bearing on the treatment selected.

STANDARD TREATMENT

The imperative need in the treatment of nephritic colic is to provide pain relief and force "passage" of the stone. This is usually accomplished with painkillers and large volumes of water, with the patient often instructed to drink up to two or three quarts per day.

The most powerful sedative used for kidney stones is morphine, but it unfortunately also has a spasm-causing effect that carries a risk of making the ureter contract, which could cause further blockage. Therefore, it is a better idea to use anti-spasmodic medications in whatever form they are available: tablets, suppositories, and shots, especially intravenously. Sometimes the doctor is even forced to put the patient on an IV to stop an excruciating and interminable attack.

Small stones (less than one centimeter) can often be broken up via an external shock wave treatment called lithotripsy. Larger stones, or stones that have been lodged for a while and may be imperiling the kidney, will require surgery.

ACUPOINT TREATMENT

Here, the role played by acupoint therapy is nothing short of brilliant. Experience shows that stimulation of the points is often far more effective than the most potent medication, and many acupuncturists can recall patients whose troubles resisted even intravenous drip, yet whose pain vanished almost immediately when needles were inserted in the appropriate points.

TECHNIQUES TO USE

Vigorous stimulation should be supplied to the points to counter a painful attack. Use deep massage or an electric stimulator until the pain vanishes. The Chinese are even known to use injections of sedatives in the appropriate points. If a stone is stuck, it is good to use the first principal point described below. Apply strong finger pressure upon it or even repeated taps from a slightly heavy object, such as a reflex hammer, which can possibly cause the kidney stone to be dislodged.

The Principal Points

The first point is located on the back, three finger-widths away from the midline, at the level of the top of the iliac crest. Stimulate the point that is on the painful side.

The second principal point is on the inside of the calf, in the notch just below the head of the tibia bone.

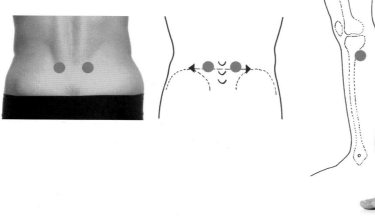

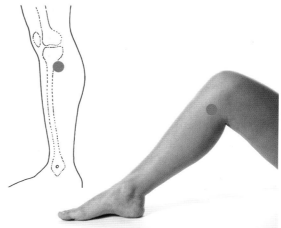

The Secondary Points

The first of these points is in the center of the back side of the calf, between the two muscle bellies located there; the second is behind the inner ankle bone, two finger-widths above the calcaneum.

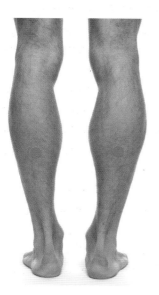

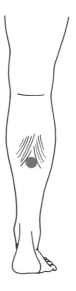

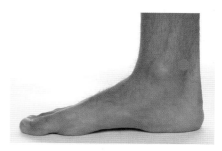

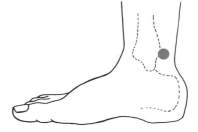

Urinary Infections, Cystitis, Pyelonephritis

URINARY INFECTIONS CAN occur anywhere along the tract that transports urine, from the kidneys to the renal pelvis, the ureter, the bladder, and the urethra. Although primary kidney infections are quite rare, infections that start elsewhere and spread to the kidneys can ultimately destroy them.

SYMPTOMS AND FORMS

The infections are different in nature depending on what area is affected. When an infection involves an attack on the upper part of the urinary apparatus (the renal pelvis and ureter), we call it pyelonephritis; when the bladder is afflicted, it is cystitis.

Pyelonephritis is always a severe infection. These cases are often acute and accompanied by high fever, intense shivering, and pain in the lumbar region. Chronic forms are less spectacular with a low-grade fever and intermittent burning sensations with urination.

This condition is most pernicious when the patient is an infant, because nothing will draw attention to the urine. Hence, the imperative obligation to have the urine examined whenever a child of nursing age exhibits a fever whose cause cannot otherwise be identified.

At all ages, it is imperative to determine the cause for an infection that manifests "upstream from a dam." In adults this dam may be due to a kidney stone or shrinkage of the ureter. In children, it is most often due to poor structure or function of the bladder, which sends the urine back up instead of allowing it to follow its natural course.

The situation is completely different with the bladder infections known as cystitis.

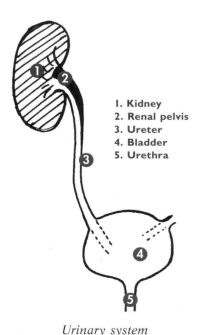

1. Kidney
2. Renal pelvis
3. Ureter
4. Bladder
5. Urethra

Urinary system

These conditions, especially in women, are infinitely less serious, though they can be a veritable scourge with their incessant repetition. Sometimes a urine examination does not even reveal the presence of any bacteria, yet the patient experiences all the symptoms of cystitis: repeated desires to urinate, burning sensation during urination, sometimes blood appears in the urine. In these cases, the affliction is called cystalgia.

CAUSES

We have already seen how an obstruction can be the primary cause for pyelonephritis.

It is not the same case for cystitis, an illness that almost exclusively strikes women, and whose origin is commonly ascribed to the proximity of the natural orifices of the female body. Germs spread out of the anus and enter the urinary tract. Clothing that is too restrictive—tight jeans, for example—can facilitate this migration, as can sexual intercourse and insufficient hygiene.

Cystalgia, meanwhile—which is a false cystitis as there are no bacteria—is usually a secondary effect of a large number of causes: allergies, neighboring genital infections, pelvis shifts, and even problems of a psychological nature.

STANDARD TREATMENT

Pyelonephritis calls for massive doses of antibiotics. Surgery is also an option for removing the obstacle at fault, which can be a tumor, a kidney stone, or something else.

On the other hand, we can say that cystitis represents the classic situation of antibiotic failure. One has only to see the numerous women suffering one relapse after another—not to mention the germ-free cystalgia—to conclude that standard medicine is not quite effective in treating these conditions.

ACUPOINT TREATMENT

While acupoint therapy is not generally used in the treatment of pyelonephritis, which requires antibiotics, it comes in first for dealing with both cystitis and cystalgia, and should be employed systematically.

TECHNIQUES TO USE

The principal and secondary points should be stimulated for a long period of time, once in the morning and once at night. Finger pressure or electrical stimulation are both options here. It is good when you can obtain a numb sensation in the area of the bladder, though this may take ten to fifteen minutes to achieve. This stimulation is a good way of avoiding critical flare-ups, and preventing any relapses—especially of cystitis.

The Principal Points

The first point is located at the bottom of the belly, on the median line just above the edge of the pubic bone. The second point is located on the back, three finger-widths away from the spine at the level of the top of the iliac crest.

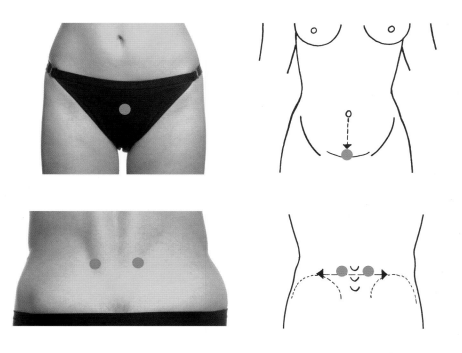

The Secondary Points

There are two secondary points. The first is located at the inside end of the knee crease; the other can be found three finger-widths away on either side of the anus.

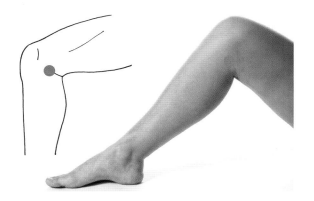

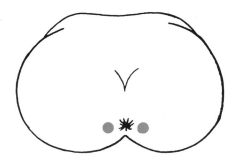

Urine Retention
and Incontinence

RETENTION OF URINE and incontinence are two diametrically opposed states: urine retention means an inability to release urine, while incontinence refers to the inability to hold it back. Interestingly, the same acupoints are used to treat both of these disorders—evidence that their action is essentially regulatory.

SYMPTOMS AND CAUSES

Retention can be an acute situation. A person can have urinated normally or with little discomfort for his whole life when suddenly one day, he experiences an abrupt halt in his ability to urinate. Though his desire to urinate remains, nothing "comes out." Quite quickly discomfort turns into pain and then becomes a real torture.

Retention can also occur in an incomplete fashion, with urine coming in dribbles or even one drip at a time. In both cases, one symptom is the same: the appearance of a "ball" in the bottom of the stomach, which is nothing other than the bladder dilated with the accumulation of urine.

When this ball is pushed upon (it is clinically known as the vesical globe), the patient's suffering will be at its maximum.

Incontinence is the complete opposite. Here, the patient is incapable of retaining his urine, which either leaks out continuously or releases in bursts after sudden movements such as coughing or laughing. This form of incontinence does not include nighttime enuresis, when children wet the bed at night, which will be discussed in the next chapter.

CAUSES

Anything that creates an obstacle to the flow of urine creates a retention. Among the most frequent causes for men are:

- Shrinking of the urethra as the result of an infection, even an old one
- Poor bladder function
- Prostatic hypertrophy, the "enlarged prostate" of elderly men

In women, the origin can be compression caused by an abdominal mass, especially a fibroid. In children, the first thing to have checked is a possible deformity of the urinary tract.

Incontinence can often be traced back to surgical or obstetrical mishaps. Among men, this is most commonly the result of a prostate operation. The incontinence is usually temporary in this case and often fixes itself, but it can, unfortunately, be permanent. Incontinence in women can also be a more or less remote consequence of childbirth. In this case it is often accompanied by a prolapse—the descent of the womb or bladder.

Finally, both incontinence and retention can be a consequence of paralysis of the spinal cord.

STANDARD TREATMENT

In cases of urine retention—especially acute ones—the first duty is to provide relief to the patient through insertion of a catheter, a kind of small semi-rigid hose that will go into the bladder and allow urine to flow out. When using a catheter is not possible, the bladder can be punctured directly through the stomach wall. But this is only an emergency measure that will allow the physician the time necessary to examine the urinary tract, by X-ray in particular, to find the precise cause and come up with the appropriate solution. This generally involves surgery.

The problem of incontinence is much harder to treat. Surgery can improve the situation sometimes by correcting any deformities or by "lifting" prolapsed organs back up, but even after this kind of operation, the results are not always complete or definitive.

ACUPOINT TREATMENT

Acupoint therapy is quite valuable in two principal cases. When acute retention is an issue, stimulation of the points can stop a spasm, allowing urine to flow and perhaps even reducing the need for catheterization. With incontinence, regular stimulation of the points can provide noticeable improvement.

TECHNIQUES TO USE

For urine retention, use finger stimulation on the points recommended below until urine appears. For incontinence, stimulate the points twice daily for fifteen minutes using finger massage or electricity. This stimulation can be usefully combined with very simple exercises of the pelvic floor known as Kegel exercises. These strengthen the muscles that hold the urine and consist of contracting and releasing the perineum for equal periods of time. To do these exercises, contract your urethra as if you were trying to stop urinating in mid-stream, hold it for one to four seconds, then release. Repeat this cycle about ten times.

The Principal Points

The first point can be found three finger-widths away and on either side of the anus; the second can be found on the lower outside corner of the little toenail.

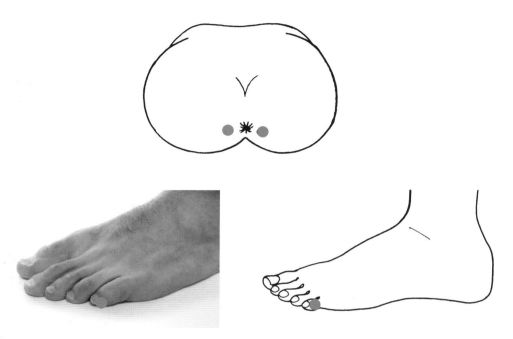

The Secondary Points

The first of the secondary points is a finger-width away from the median line, at the level of the pubic bone; the second is a finger-width below those points, slightly to the outside.

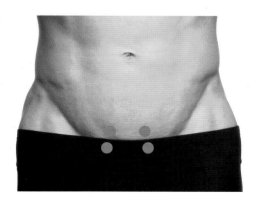

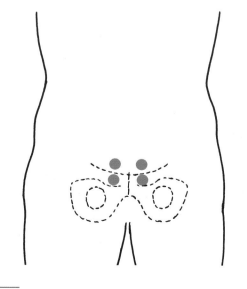

Pediatric Bedwetting

NIGHTTIME CONTINENCE—IN OTHER words, no longer wetting the bed—is something that is normally established between the ages of two and three years old. But it is perfectly acceptable for accidents to happen every now and then until a child is five or six.

It is futile and even risky to demand continence of a child who is younger than two or three. Some parents are perfect maniacs when it comes to toilet-training and literally persecute their babies trying to get them to use the "potty." This is an irrational attitude and unfortunately one that can have a long-lasting disturbing effect on the child.

There are two types of nocturnal bedwetting. *Primary enuresis* refers to a child who has continuously wet the bed—in other words, one who has never been fully toilet-trained. *Secondary enuresis* refers to a child who toilet-trained in the normal fashion, then started wetting the bed again two or three years later. This secondary symptom can occur in reaction to an emotional shock, like the birth of a little brother or sister, the separation of the parents, and so on.

Enuresis of either kind amounts to a significant impairment, however: the child will feel embarrassed and ashamed around his friends; he or she may not be able to go to summer camp or spend the night at a friend's house. This will eventually leave some kind of mark on the personality and make the child very unhappy.

CAUSES

There are two major causes of enuresis. Psychological cases are the first to be cited. And it is true that they play a predominant role—the examples cited above for secondary enuresis can attest to that.

On the other hand, physical causes often are the dominant origin in cases of primary enuresis. The bladder may be deformed in some cases, or its contractions are too strong, or it may be because—for unknown reasons—the bladder is too small and not growing in proportion with the child. In addition, some children sleep quite soundly, and simply don't wake up when their bladder is full.

Bedwetting has no serious physiological repercussions—it just simply goes on and on. The years go by while the little "invalid" and his or her parents despair. Often it is necessary to wait until puberty before everything resolves. Sometimes the impairment lasts until adulthood, however, with all the social consequences that this entails.

STANDARD TREATMENT

From the explanation of the causes, it is easy to deduce that this treatment will consist of two parts: one psychological, the other physiological.

Psychological treatment remains the most important and is not easy to conduct. It primarily involves training or retraining the child's reflexes by prompting him to urinate at set times during the day, and to wake up one or two times a night to urinate as well. Simple alarm systems are readily available that wake a child up when they detect even a small amount of urine. The child then learns to recognize the feeling of a full bladder. At the same time, it is also necessary to play down the importance of the situation both with the child and the parents, by encouraging them to realize that the condition is not abnormal, dirty, or something to feel guilty or ashamed about. This requires a lot of tact and perseverance.

Fairly recently, medications have been used to address the physical component of the symptom. They can be effective in many cases, but only for as long as they are used. When the medication is discontinued, the wetting often resumes.

ACUPOINT TREATMENT

With an affliction this capricious and upsetting, it is difficult to predict with certainty what results will be obtained in any particular case. In my experience, I would say that favorable results will occur about 50 percent of the time, which is not so bad.

TECHNIQUES TO USE

It is necessary to stimulate each of the points for about a dozen minutes in the evening before bedtime. The result you are looking for is a numb sensation in the genital area. In China, they even use injections of vitamins or placental extract at these points.

The Principal Points

The first point is located on the inner side of the calf, a hand-width above the ankle, in a small hollow on the back edge of the tibia. The second is located on the lower abdomen, halfway between the navel and the pubic bone.

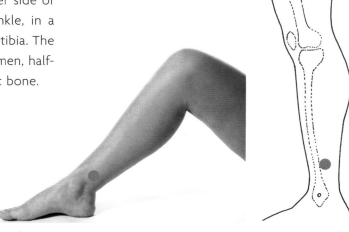

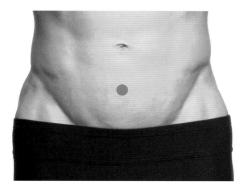

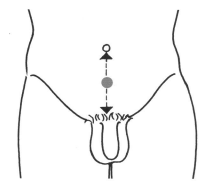

The Secondary Points

The first of these points is located on the very top of the head at the intersection of the median line with a line going from one ear to the other. The second point is on the inside of the calf, a hand-width below the knee, in the notch just below the head of the tibia.

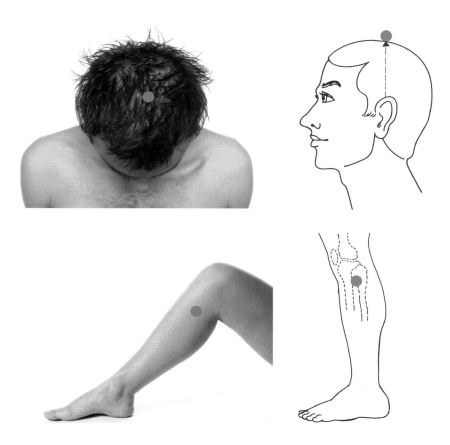

PART SEVEN

Pain

Headache

HEADACHES CAN APPEAR in a large variety of places, affecting the entire head, or just the temples, the forehead, the eyes, the neck, and so forth. They also come in a wide variety of forms: throbbing pain, burning pain, dull pain, or its opposite, "splitting" pain.

Headaches can also be accompanied by numerous complications, including a stuffy nose and dizzy spells, but especially nausea and vomiting. (This is likely the basis for the famous "liver crisis"—so dear to the French—which actually never existed for the simple reason that the head is causing the liver and bile ducts to suffer and not the reverse.)

But there is one particular headache that stands out from all the rest: the true migraine. According to recent statistics, 25 percent of the population is affected by migraines. It is easy to see the kind of repercussions this can have socially and economically.

Migraines are a hereditary disorder that generally affect one half of the head. They are often accompanied by visual symptoms and digestive problems. They can occur unexpectedly or follow a specific rhythm (which is the case with the menstrual migraines suffered by women).

CAUSES

Migraines aside, it could be said that most health problems—from fever to simple exhaustion—are accompanied by some kind of headache. It is therefore always necessary to clarify that the trouble is not related to a local cause such as eyestrain or an infection of the sinuses, teeth, or ears. Some headaches are caused by the displacement of a vertebra in the nape of the neck. This can trigger several kinds of headache, including migraines.

Finally, Americans give pride of place here to psychological pains and stress. It may be that this holds the same place for Americans as the "liver crisis" does for the French.

STANDARD TREATMENT

The treatments offered by conventional medicine are unfortunately all based on the use of pharmaceutical products. These are toxic and become dangerous when taken repeatedly.

ACUPOINT TREATMENT

This therapy should be the treatment of first resort. Generally speaking it is quite effective on all kinds of head pain and has no disadvantages.

TECHNIQUES TO USE

Massage the corresponding points quite strongly during a headache, until the pain vanishes. Electrical stimulation is preferable in these cases. There is one general point to be used for all kinds of headaches, and an assortment of others to choose from, depending on the location of the pain.

The points can also be used preventively: stimulate them for several minutes in the morning and in the evening. In this way, you can lengthen the interval between migraines and reduce the symptoms, if not banish them outright. For women with cyclical migraines related to the menstrual cycle, be sure to begin the massages at least two weeks before you expect a headache.

The Principal Point

One point can be used for all cases: it is located on the back of the head in a little notch at the edge of the occiput, three finger-widths from the auricle of the ear. Vigorous massage of this point will cause a sensation of numbness that will gradually take over the entire head and drive the pain away. But this point should always be stimulated in combination with one of the points below.

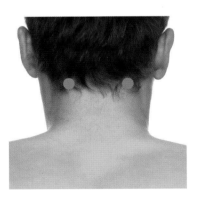

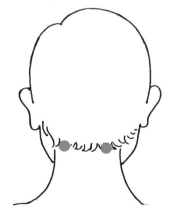

The Secondary Points

If the headache occurs in the forehead and temples, the point to stimulate is located on the palm side of the wrist, a bit below the crease, in the spot where you can feel the beat of the radial pulse.

If the headache is on the top of the head, the point to stimulate is located on the outside of the calf, a hand-width above the tip of the ankle.

If the headache affects the area around the nape of the neck, its corresponding point is located on the side of the hand beneath the little finger, at the top end of the life line. This point has a contralateral effect: stimulate the point on the left hand for a pain on the right side of the neck and vice versa.

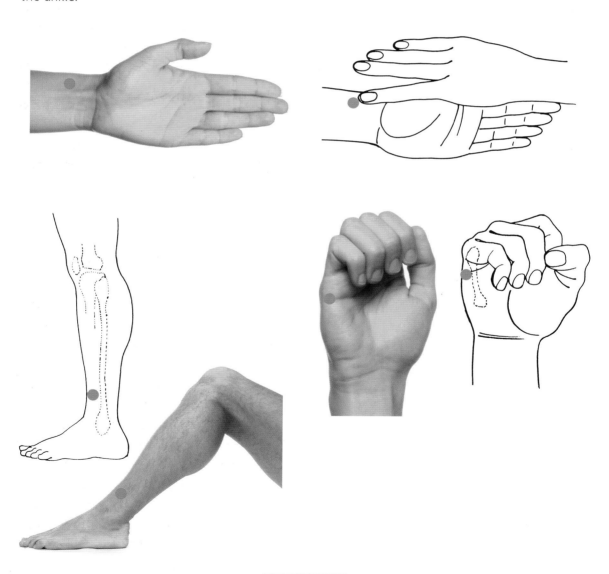

Facial Pain

DISORDERS OF THE teeth, nose, and sinus can reveal their presence through facial pain, but the most specific form of facial pain is the facial neuralgia connected to an affliction of the trigeminal nerve.

This nerve, which provides the face with its sensitivity, is divided into three branches that come to the surface of the skin at three points placed in an almost vertical line—next to the inner end of the eyebrow, beneath the eye, and on the side of the chin. Each of these three points can be affected by disease, as can all of them at once.

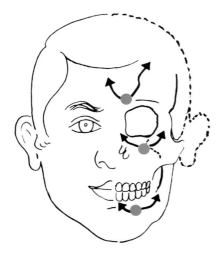

The three branches of the trigeminal nerve with the skin zones affected by each.

In its typical form, facial neuralgia cannot be mistaken for anything else. It comes on suddenly like a flash of lightning, or like the flash from a camera, and follows the course traced by the trigger zone on the cheek, the gums, or the nose. The pain only lasts for a few seconds, but what a few seconds! It prevents the individual from eating or brushing his teeth, even from talking or laughing. There is no pain in between attacks as a general rule, though the attacks can occur in quick succession.

In some cases the pain is less intense but continuous, and is often accompanied by facial flushing.

CAUSES

It is no use looking for the cause of facial neuralgia in the sinuses or the teeth. (In fact, far too many teeth have been extracted from neuralgia sufferers in an attempt to stop the pain.) It's usually quite difficult to pinpoint the exact cause, which is most likely an inflammation or virus that attacked the nerve somewhere along its course.

An eye should be kept out for the possible appearance of a case of shingles. It will make its presence known with a rash on the area of skin above the nerve endings.

In general, facial neuralgia remains depressingly similar in its effects for years on end, with phases of dormancy and phases where it is aggravated to such an extent it can lead a patient to contemplate suicide.

STANDARD TREATMENT

Regular sedatives do not relieve the pains of facial neuralgia, but anti-convulsive medications are usually effective. They are quite toxic, however, with many side effects, and their effectiveness diminishes sharply with regular use. Sometimes surgery is recommended.

ACUPOINT TREATMENT

Acupoint therapy is truly effective in cases of facial pain, and offers no danger. It is there-fore of great value in countering this disease and its sudden attacks.

TECHNIQUES TO USE

Stimulation of the points is extremely help-ful during pain flashes when there is no other recourse at hand—except your hand. Massage the points until the pain decreases. Furthermore, persistent stimulation of the points several times a day should do a great deal for reducing the intensity of the attacks and lengthening the intervals between them. For this treatment, stimulate the appropriate points for ten minutes in the morning and in the evening, every other day.

The Principal Point

There is one principal point. It is located on the palm side of the wrist, a bit beneath the crease, at the place where the radial pulse is felt.

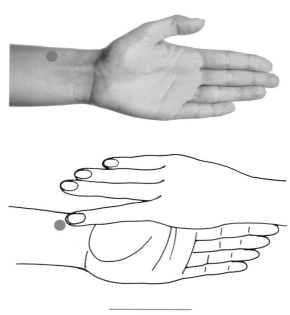

The Secondary Points

These points are located at the ends of the three branches of the nerve. For an attack on the first branch of the trigeminal nerve, stimulate the points on the inside end of the eyebrows; for the second branch, the points are just beneath the eye in the center of the orbit. For the third branch, the points are located on the chin, two finger-widths away on either side of the median line.

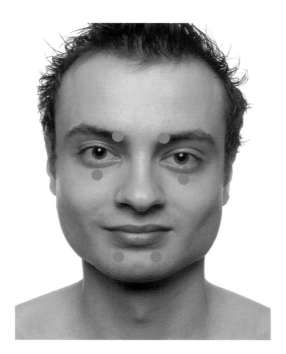

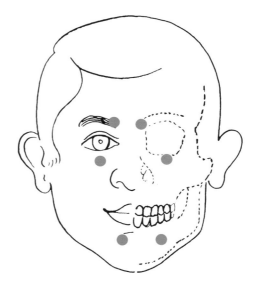

Chest Pain, Intercostal Neuralgia

PAINS IN THE chest can be quite varied, ranging from a simple "stitch in the side" to a crushing pain that affects the entire thorax. Pain can overflow into the neck or stomach, or radiate into the nape or along an arm. The type of pain depends largely upon the cause. Intercostal neuralgia is typically accompanied by a burning sensation along one of the ribs, which can extend into the back or stomach.

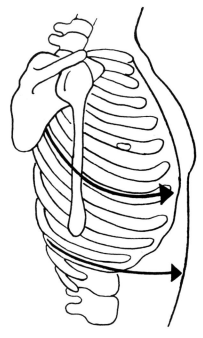

Intercostal neuralgia: pain along the lower ribs can "spill over" into the stomach.

CAUSES

The causes of chest pain are also many and diverse. The simple stitch in the side is due to violent contraction of the spleen following a muscular effort (the athletes of ancient Greece had this organ removed, hence the old expression in many European countries, "to run like you have no spleen").

But chest pains often have a much more dire meaning: they can be caused by problems of the heart, lungs, or pleura. Spasms in the coronary arteries cause angina pectoralis, whose typical form is a band of crushing pain across the thorax that travels down the left arm.

In intercostal neuralgia, a band of pain half circles the chest. It can be due to a fractured rib or an eruptive disease: shingles, whose most frequent location is on the chest. This can also be due simply to a displaced rib that has pinched an intercostal nerve, whose pain will echo into the chest.

STANDARD TREATMENT

Standard treatment is quite different depending on the cause of the pain; treatments for the more serious forms of chest pain will not be covered here. On the other hand, pain due to shingles, cracked ribs, or intercostal neuralgia have practically no standard treatment options outside of sedatives and analgesics.

ACUPOINT TREATMENT

Acupoint therapy has no peer when it comes to dealing with a neuralgia caused by shingles, a costal crack, or a pain of vertebral origin. Especially since standard treatment options are so limited, acupoint therapy should be pursued for any of these ailments.

TECHNIQUES TO USE

The points to stimulate should be on the same side as the pain. The intensity of the stimulation will vary depending on the cause. Electrical stimulation is ideal for shingles, but a vigorous massage can also be quite effective. A single session should suffice, as long as the stimulation lasts until the pain disappears.

For chronic pains, it is a good idea to stimulate the points for several minutes in the morning and in the evening.

The Principal Point

The principal point is on the back of the forearm, directly in the center. Find the spot along the centerline that is most tender when pressed.

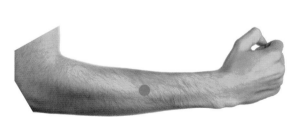

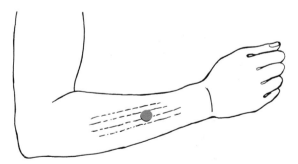

The Secondary Points

There are two secondary points: one is located on the tip of the last (twelfth) rib, the floating side. It can be found by tracing your finger down along the side of the rib cage until you reach the bottom rib.

The second point is on the inside of the leg, beneath the knee, in the notch just beneath the head of the tibia bone.

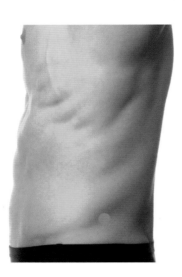

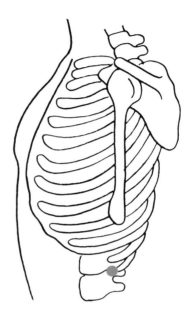

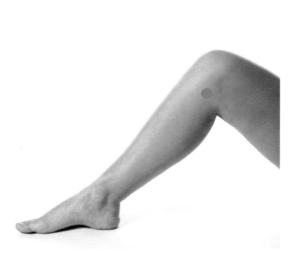

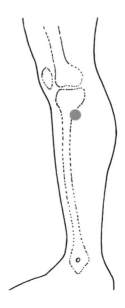

PART EIGHT

Skin and Dermatological Problems

Chilblains

CHILBLAINS, WHICH IS sometimes mistaken for frostbite, are small superficial ulcerations that can affect the extremities of the body when they're exposed to cold.

They begin as gleaming and painful reddish blotches, which generally occur during the winter. The lesions can remain in this state, or they can ulcerate and secrete blood and fluid. At this stage they can form into one large lesion—along the entire edge of the ear, for example, or the circumference of the heel. The pain they cause at this point can be quite substantial, preventing ordinary movements, the wearing of shoes, and so forth. The lesions will often close up spontaneously without treatment, leaving behind a whitish network of scarring. In susceptible people, this process may begin all over again with the coming of the next winter.

CAUSES

Chilblains are due to the inflammation of the small capillaries beneath the skin. When chilled skin is suddenly warmed—next to a heater or by a fire, for instance—the capillaries can expand more quickly than surrounding arteries, causing a leakage of blood into nearby tissues. Dietary deficiencies also play a large role here.

STANDARD TREATMENT

The best treatment is prevention: protection against the cold for the specific areas of the body most at risk of chilblains. In addition, the B vitamin niacin or blood vessel dilators are sometimes prescribed.

ACUPOINT TREATMENT

This therapy brings about an immediate calming of the pain. It also lengthens the time between relapses, and can prevent the appearance of new chilblains.

TECHNIQUES TO USE

For relief of acute pain, massage these points from three to four minutes, and also massage the circumference of each chilblain.

As a preventive measure, massage the points for two to three minutes once in the morning and once at night, starting at the beginning of winter.

The Principal Point

The principal point is located in the nape of the neck, beneath the seventh cervical verte-bra. When the head is tilted slightly forward, the seventh cervical vertebra will usually "bump out" visibly.

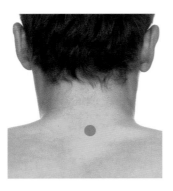 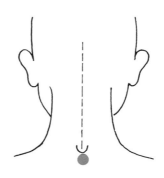

The Secondary Points

The first secondary point is located on the very top of the head at the intersection of the median line with a line going from one ear to the other; the second is on the sole of the foot, in the hollow that is formed when the toes curl in.

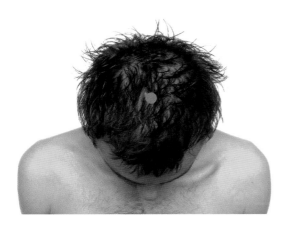 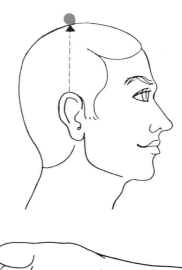

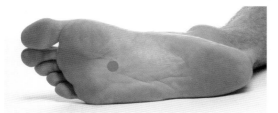 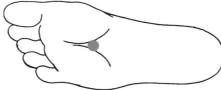

Eczema

ECZEMA, ALSO CALLED dermatitis, is a family of skin diseases characterized by a permanent red eruption, generally covered by tiny blisters called vesicles. These lesions tend to itch ferociously. A person may have a tiny patch of eczema somewhere, or a generalized eczema that can cover almost the entire body. Some locations are particularly annoying, like those that involve the face, for example, or particularly painful, like those that attack the genital regions.

Eczema lesions can be dry, cracked, and crusty, or completely opposite: oozing a yellowish fluid. They can become infected or, conversely become sclerotic. This is frequently the case with the worsening of this condition known as lichenified eczema. The patient's skin has a leathery barklike appearance at this stage of the disease.

In all cases, there is one point in common: the itching, which—depending on the seriousness of the eruption—can go from a passing inconvenience to a never-ending torture that can even pose a threat to the mental stability of the afflicted individual.

CAUSES

While there are a half-dozen varieties of eczema, the most common forms are allergic contact eczema and atopic eczema. In allergic contact eczema, also called contact dermatitis, the skin becomes sensitized to contact with a particular material—most often a chemical substance like cement, household cleaning products, leather, rubber, cosmetics (eyeliner, fingernail polish), or a plant or animal substance (cat fur, and so on). Whenever the patient touches this material, he or she develops the characteristic rash. Often it attacks a specific region—the face or hands, for example. The vast growth in the number of chemical products today has brought along with it a veritable explosion in the number of allergic contact eczema cases.

Atopic eczema does not require physical contact with an allergen to produce a rash. Environmental allergens may be a factor in its development, as the condition often co-occurs with asthma and allergies. Most often it is hereditary, and can appear in infancy.

Lastly, it should be pointed out that any skin disease can cause an eczema outbreak.

STANDARD TREATMENT

The first step in treating allergic contact eczema is to try to determine the triggering cause and remove it from the patient's environment. Sometimes allergists will undertake a program of progressive desensitization to the allergens using weekly injections.

This is a long and often disappointing task, however, because there are frequently several allergens involved. Just as the patient's sensitivity to one allergen has been adjusted, he will often become acutely sensitive to another product.

With atopic eczema, the most common treatment strategy is to try and calm the inflammation: the best known sedative in this regard is cortisone and its derivatives, administered topically, orally, or by injection.

But this can be a dreadful weapon. Its use is certainly often followed by spectacular improvement, but it is also subsequently followed in most cases by a dangerous "rebound" after the treatment has stopped. The treatment, moreover, is one that can cause all manner of complications.

ACUPOINT TREATMENT

The nature of this condition is so diverse that it is often difficult to talk about a cure, but any treatment that can provide even a modicum of relief is well worth trying. Acupoint therapy can ease the symptoms of an acute flare-up of eczema or provide gradual improvement to a chronic case.

TECHNIQUES TO USE

Vigorously stimulate the points for several minutes when treating an acute rash. Repeat the stimulation as often as necessary.

Chronic eruptions, on the other hand, require massages several times a day for five to ten minutes at a time, or the use of electrical stimulation.

The Principal Points

There are two principal points that should be stimulated in all cases of eczema.

The first is located on the back, two finger-widths on either side of the third thoracic vertebra. (See page 9 for instructions on locating this point.)

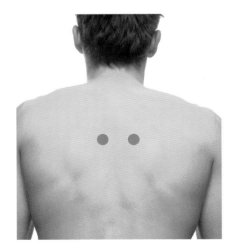
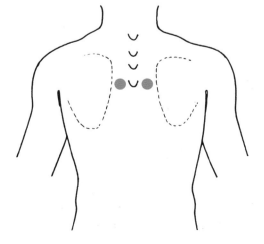

The Principal Points (continued)

The second principal point is on the back of the knee, in the center of the crease.

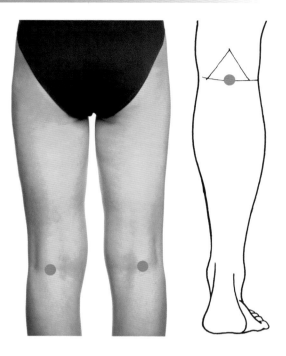

The Secondary Points

The two secondary points will reinforce the effect of the principal points in chronic and tenacious cases of this disease.

The first of these points is on the outside end of the elbow crease. The second point is on the front of the thigh: place your palm over the kneecap with your fingers spread; the thumb will indicate the correct location of the point.

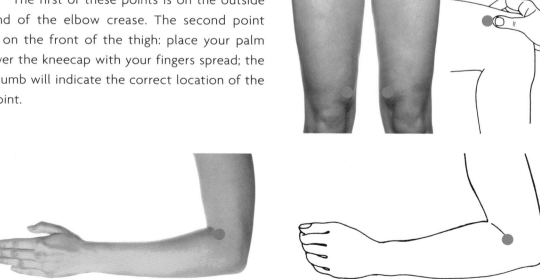

Hives

HIVES (URTICARIA) IS a rash consisting of red, pink, or white elements that disappear under pressure. This is a very important point: the spots go away when pushed on but reappear immediately when the pressure is released. This is how they can be distinguished from other skin eruptions such as eczema.

Hives are terribly irritating. The sensation they cause is a stinging throbbing tautness that is an annoyance day and night.

FORMS

There are allergic and chronic forms of the ailment. In addition to patches of hives, which are the most common presentation, there are giant hives that cover the entire body when the patches merge into a single mass. In the condition called Quincke's edema, the face may become deformed by large hives until it looks like an inflating balloon.

CAUSES

Ordinary hives occur as a reaction to a foreign product like a medication, a food, or an insect sting. It is the quintessential form of allergy-caused illness.

Chronic urticaria has less clear causes. There may be factors in the intercellular environment that have yet to be completely determined.

STANDARD TREATMENT

The conventional treatment for hives is anti-allergy medications, primarily antihistamines. Sometimes doctors will feel forced to resort to cortisone and derivative medications.

ACUPOINT TREATMENT

Acupoint therapy is valuable here, both in the treatment of an acute crisis and for attempting to improve a chronic condition. I think that it is always something that should be used from the start. In the event it does not work, or not sufficiently, one can always turn to the standard medications.

TECHNIQUES TO USE

When treating an acute case of hives, stimulate the requisite points for two to three minutes every half hour.

For chronic urticaria, stimulate the points for ten minutes in the morning and again at night. This is a situation where electrical stimulation is preferable.

The Principal Points

The first point is located between the shoulder blades, two finger-widths away on either side of the third thoracic vertebra (See page 9 for guidelines on finding this vertebra.) The second point is located in the middle of the knee crease.

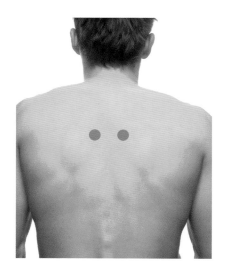

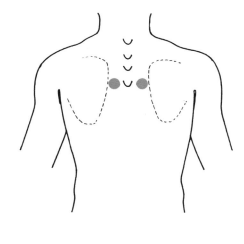

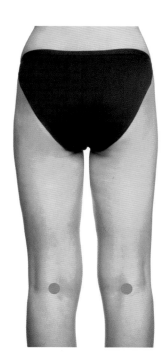

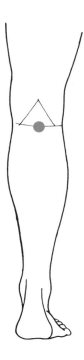

The Secondary Points

The first secondary point is located on the outside end of the elbow crease; the second point is right at the middle of the bottom edge of the skull.

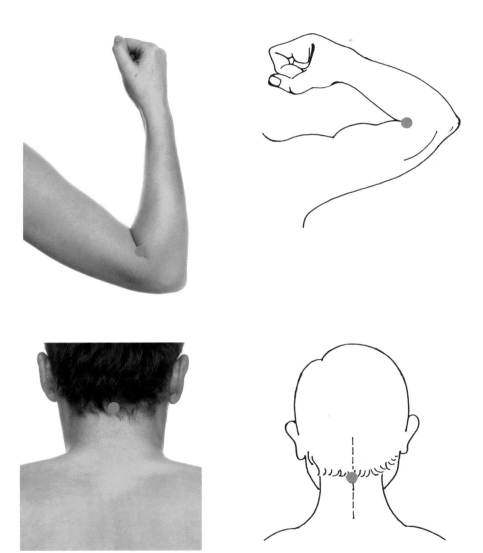

Shingles, Chicken Pox, and Herpes

ALL THREE OF these diseases are caused by related viruses. The symptom they all share is the appearance of an often severe rash on the skin.

SYMPTOMS AND FORMS

Shingles is a very odd affliction. It manifests along the course of a nerve and reveals it presence by the appearance of a blister-filled rash and red patches at various spots along this nerve's trajectory. This eruption is accompanied by fever and pain that can be stinging, stabbing, or throbbing. It can happen that even when the visible signs of the illness have subsided, the pain can persist for months and even years. This can make the life of the sufferer quite miserable.

As there are nerves everywhere beneath the skin, shingles can "emerge" anywhere on the body, but it only does so in a unilateral fashion. You can have shingles on your left side or your right side, but not on both sides. The most frequent site for it is the thorax, along the intercostal nerve. The illness will appear as a series of rashes on one half of the chest, with two patches on the back, one on the side, and one or two on the breast.

But shingles can appear at other spots on the body including the face. One of the most dangerous forms of this disease is ophthalmic shingles, which causes rashes on the scalp and forehead but whose seriousness lies in the fact that it can reach into the eyes with all the risks that entails: keratitis, ocular tears, residual leicoma.

Why place chicken pox—a benign disease if ever there was one—in the company of shingles? Because it is the same disease. An individual infected with shingles can give chicken pox to the children with whom he enters into contact. It is believed that the varicella virus will become fixed in a nerve and can cause relapses in the form of shingles when the individual is an adult.

Chicken pox in children also appears in the form of a blistery rash, but one that can appear anywhere on the skin and mucous membranes and develop for a period of fifteen days to three weeks during which time it may have several acute flare-ups.

Herpes, meanwhile, can be described as

a miniature case of shingles. Only one or two patches of the rash appear on the skin or mucous membranes.

But herpes always comes back (often when the patient has a fever, or during a menstrual period), and the relapse always occurs at the same spot—most commonly the lips, nose, and/or buttocks. Two locations that are particularly painful are the genital organs (both male and female) and the eye, for which the dangers are the same as for ophthalmic shingles.

What's more, genital herpes in a pregnant woman can infect the newborn and cause serious cerebral problems (encephalitis).

CAUSES

We saw earlier that these three diseases are caused by various strains of virus: the varicella virus and at least two varieties of the herpes virus.

STANDARD TREATMENT

An assortment of antiviral medications have some effect on the most serious forms of herpes and shingles, but these products are fairly toxic and not all people's bodies will support their use.

ACUPOINT TREATMENT

If I may say so, shingles is the triumph of acupuncture. The consistency of results and the speed of action still are cause for surprise, even among experienced practitioners. Acupressure massage and electrical stimulation are also quite effective.

TECHNIQUES TO USE

The massage should be vigorous to truly stimulate these points:

- either a strong massage lasting half an hour or longer,
- or intense electrical stimulation.

It is not unusual to see the patient—who had been going through torture before the session—leave completely soothed, and to see the rash dry up and disappear within the next twenty-four hours.

The Points

Point selection depends on the location of the lesion. I have spelled out the three most frequent situations.

For *intercostal shingles,* the principal point is located on the top of the forearm, midway between the wrist crease and the inner side of the elbow crease, in the hollow between the two bones; its secondary points are located on the side of the little toe, on the corner of the toenail and at its base, against the joint.

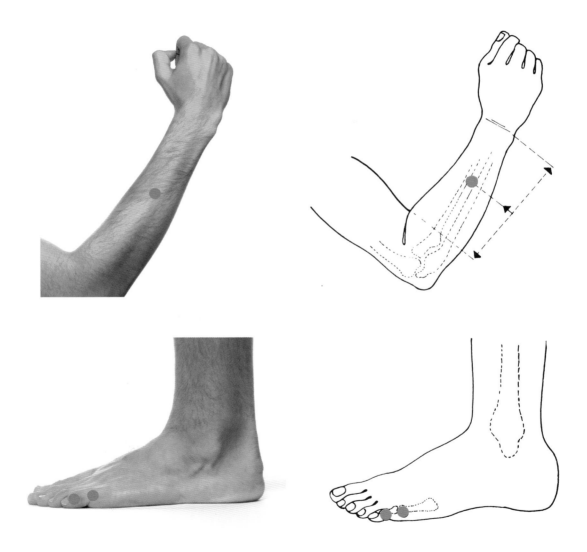

For *ophthalmic shingles* or herpes the first point is on the hand, in the notch formed by the junction of the index finger and the thumb; the other point is at the end of the second toe, on the lower outside corner of the nail.

For *chicken pox* the first point described for intercostal shingles is the principal point to stimulate here; it is located at the midpoint of the forearm between the edges of the arm and the elbow and wrist crease.

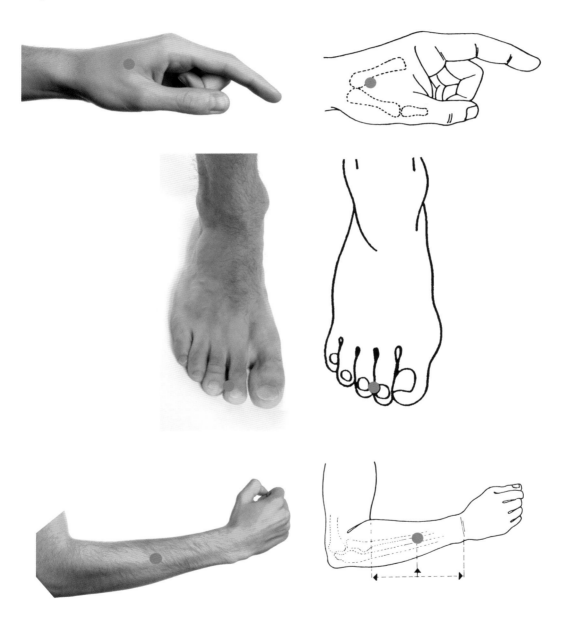

The Points (continued)

There are two secondary points: one is on the nape of the neck in a small hollow at the edge of the skull, two finger-widths away from the auricle of the ear; the other is at the base of the second toe, on the side nearer the big toe.

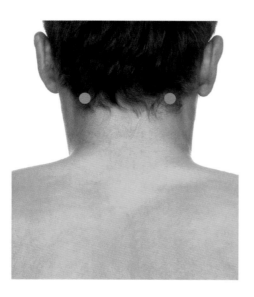

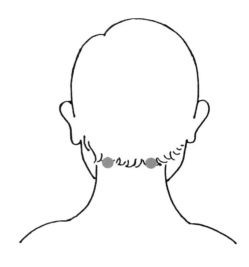

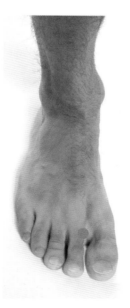

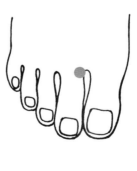

Psoriasis

THE CHARACTERISTIC SYMPTOM of psoriasis—as well as other diseases with "dry" eruptions—is a more or less circular rough red patch covered with "scabs" that can be peeled off. These scabs form numerous small patches of skin known as squama or scales.

Most often the lesions appear as isolated patches, which tend to be on the large side. As a rule, they don't sting, but more severe cases can be itchy and/or painful. Sometimes the patches spread and merge together, almost covering the entire body. This sufferer will constantly be shedding scales, which can be found in his clothes and bedding.

Sometimes psoriasis affects only one part of the body, such as the palms of the hand and the soles of the feet, or the scalp (this is one of the rare forms of the disease that itches), or it can even destroy the nails. When it takes these forms diagnosis can be difficult because it can resemble other skin diseases (lichen planus, for example). A severe form of psoriasis is psoriatic arthritis, which is accompanied by arthritic joint pain—usually in the hands and fingers.

Generally speaking, psoriasis is a lifelong disease with phases of remission and renewed outbreaks. While it is sometimes discreet, it can have a detrimental effect on the life of the afflicted individual who may feel reluctant to go to the beach or to get undressed around other people.

CAUSES

The causes of this disease are not known with any certainty. For some, outbreaks can be connected to infections or psychological shocks, or they can fall into the context of autoimmune disease.

STANDARD TREATMENT

There is no specific treatment. If there are not many patches and they are spread far apart, a local treatment using creams with a coal tar or cortisone base is possible. If the psoriasis is extensive, a general treatment is required. Ultraviolet light treatments are effective, especially when combined with substances called *psoralens*, which improve the body's sensitivity to light.

ACUPOINT TREATMENT

What are the results offered by our therapy? They are very uneven. However, it is true that it is difficult to come to a clear opinion when it comes to diseases whose development is so capricious. The treatment is worth trying, as it is frequently effective.

TECHNIQUES TO USE

To combat an affliction as tenacious as this, perseverance is the key. Using finger massage, repeat the stimulations two or three times a day for ten to fifteen minutes at a time. Using an electronic method to provide more continuous stimulation is also worth trying. This is one way you may bring an end to a flare-up of the disease and thereby improve the patient's mental state.

The Principal Points

The first principal point is at the outer end of the elbow crease. The second point is on the front of the thigh: place your palm over the kneecap with your fingers spread; your thumb will indicate the correct location.

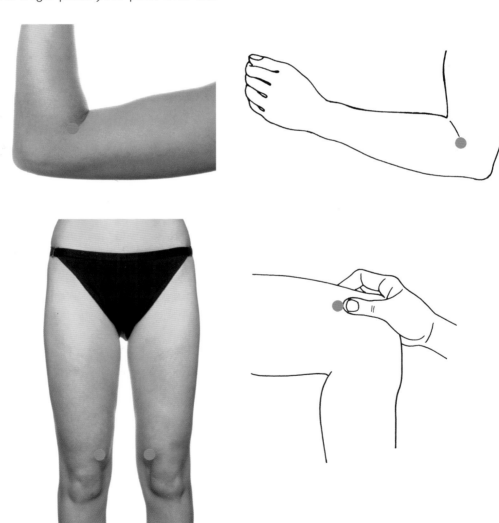

The Secondary Points

Massage toward the psoriasis patch from the four cardinal directions (see illustration at right).

For patches on the face and scalp: use a point located on the underside of the forearm, where the pulse can be felt, a few finger-widths below the wrist crease.

For patches on the palms of the hands and nails, use the point located on the back of the wrist just below the point where the two arm bones meet.

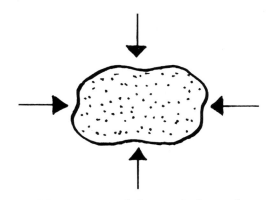

Massage toward the psoriasis patch

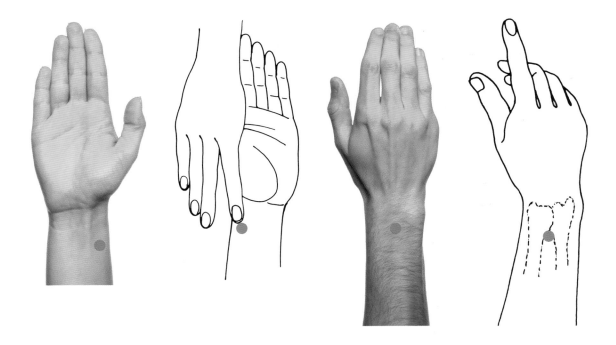

The Secondary Points (continued)

For patches on the feet: use the point located on the top of the foot, directly in the center—halfway between both sides and halfway between the two ends.

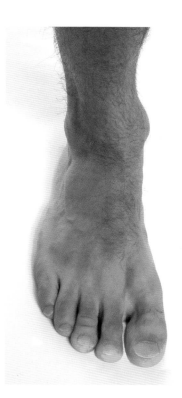
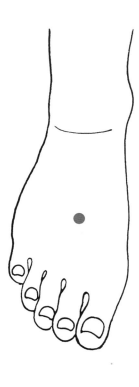

PART NINE

Respiratory Ailments

Asthma

ASTHMA IS A disease of the bronchial tubes, characterized by episodes of labored breathing that is particularly evident on exhalation.

Generally, asthma attacks occur in rather abrupt fashion at night, around two or three o'clock in the morning. The patient will be awoken by an uncontrollable coughing fit, followed by a desperate "thirst" for air. He will sit on his bed, clutching at objects. His neck will swell and his eyes bulge from his head, the hiss of his breath and the puffing out of his chest will reveal the efforts he is making to breathe. After a period of time, the crisis will diminish. The patient may then spit a little before falling back in total exhaustion. This is a typical asthma attack.

But often asthma does not appear in its pure form like this. Sometimes the subject exhibits less violent distress but the attacks last longer. This is usually the case with older asthma sufferers, for whom dyspnea has become a near-permanent condition.

Asthma attacks can be severe enough to be life-threatening.

CAUSES

Not all respiratory distress (clinically known as dyspnea) is asthma. Dyspnea can be caused by the larynx, the heart, or other pulmonary diseases. Only a doctor will be able to tell the difference.

The more asthma itself is studied, however, the more complex it appears, and the greater the number of causes detected for it. In addition to the allergic causes, which are manifold, a large place must now be given to the infectious asthma that is often a side effect of bronchial infections. Hereditary factors play a large role in the development of asthma, and for chronic sufferers, emotional reactions are known to contribute to attacks.

STANDARD TREATMENT

The many different causes of asthma and the various mechanics involved have brought about the use of a huge number of medications. These can be divided into several categories:

- Theophylline and its derivatives; these medications, which have long been used in the treatment of asthma, continue to be a first line of defense
- Cortisone in various forms
- Adrenaline derivatives
- Lastly, a number of new substances that are too varied to be successfully described here

All of these substances can be administered as shots, suppositories, pills, or inhalants. In addition to their beneficial properties, however, all of these medications can have dangerous effects. Only a doctor or other trained medical professional should be allowed to prescribe them—and always at the minimum effective dose. Be on the lookout to prevent any excessive self-medication!

ACUPOINT TREATMENT

Acupoint therapy can prove helpful to asthma sufferers in two ways:

- For immediate use during an asthma attack, where it can relieve discomfort and reduce its duration

- With repeated or continuous stimulation in treatment of chronic asthma, the results are often positive and this method has no drawbacks

TECHNIQUES TO USE

During a severe asthma attack, stimulate the principal points until the crisis subsides and the patient expectorates. Finger massage should be especially vigorous for this treatment.

To treat chronic asthma, stimulate the points for five minutes two or three times a day, or use an electrical stimulator to provide continuous stimulation.

The Principal Points

The first point is located on the back, two finger-widths on either side of the third thoracic vertebra. To find this spot, find the vertebral projection at the nape as described on page 9 and count three beneath it.

The second principal point is on the sternum between the two breasts.

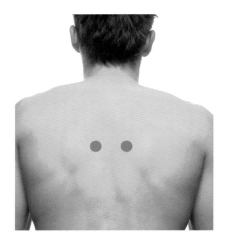
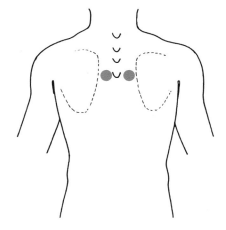

The Principal Points (continued)

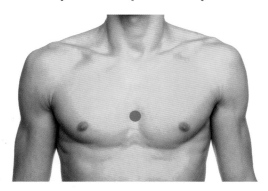 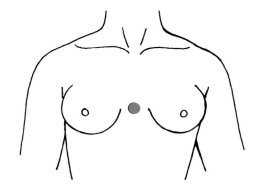

The Secondary Points

The first point is located on the tip of the Adam's apple; the second is on the outer calf, two finger-widths above the midpoint between the ankle and the knee. This point is very valuable for dealing with excessive quantities of expectoration.

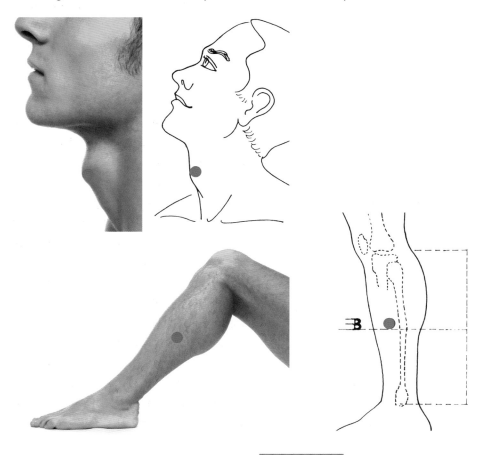

Bronchitis

BRONCHITIS IS THE clinical term for infection of the bronchial tubes. It is characterized by a cough that usually begins as a dry cough, which becomes chestier and wetter as the ailment progresses.

The expectorations only appear later in the disease's development. They are first a purulent yellow or green, then become white when the illness reaches the end of its development.

FORMS

A clear distinction needs to be drawn between acute bronchitis and the chronic form of the ailment. Acute bronchitis is what follows a banal cold or flu. The patient's fever rises and breathing becomes difficult, often with a burning feeling. The patient will have coughing fits, and eventually will expectorate phlegm. Normally, with or without treatment, this disease will resolve itself in two to three weeks. After this time the individual will be basically cured and have no after-effects to deal with.

But it is an entirely different story with chronic bronchitis. In this case, the patient starts coughing in autumn and frankly never stops. A copious quantity of expectoration continues throughout this time. The disease then returns in full force with fever and coughing, the expectorations become purulent, and the patient spends the entire winter going from one relapse to the next.

But this is not merely an annoying indisposition; it is an extremely serious disease that is one of the major causes of death in modern times. The individual's respiratory capacity diminishes, and the heart eventually becomes seriously impaired, leaving the patient vulnerable to many life-threatening complications. Every step must be taken to avoid this disastrous evolution.

CAUSES

While acute bronchitis is connected to an infection of the respiratory tract by one of the countless germs that normally live inside it, chronic bronchitis requires a particular set of circumstances to develop.

Among these circumstances I would like to single out two in particular: the dilation of the bronchia and tobacco. The dilation of the bronchial tubes is often a disorder acquired at birth or during childhood, as the result of whooping cough or the numerous cases of rhinopharyngitis that are the sorry privilege of children growing up in cities. Because the bronchial tubes are too flabby, they are incapable of expelling secretions, which instead sit there stagnating and going septic.

Among adults, it is vital to stress what a disastrous role the primary pollutant tobacco plays here. This is at least something that everyone has the power to change if they so wish.

STANDARD TREATMENT

Acute bronchitis is the exact type of disease antibiotics were designed to treat. They generally have good results here, but they also include the digestive disadvantages and other complications that can result from using these medications. Treating chronic bronchitis is again a whole different story. It requires an entire group of therapies to use either successively or at the same time: antibiotics, corticoids, heart tonics, and even oxygen. Lifelong antibiotic treatment is now recognized as too dangerous and consequently it has been abandoned. Breathing exercises, on the other hand, are always helpful and harmless.

ACUPOINT TREATMENT

Acupoint therapy provides different treatments for the acute and chronic forms of bronchitis. In the case of acute bronchitis, the treatment should be applied as soon as possible at the beginning of the illness to stop it completely or at least reduce its duration. In chronic cases, acupoint therapy is one of numerous means that can be used to stabilize the patient's condition, and as always, it has no dangerous side effects. It offers valuable help for respiratory therapy.

TECHNIQUES TO USE

What's called for in the treatment of acute bronchitis is vigorous manual stimulation every half hour or every hour as soon as possible after the onset of the disease. Chronic bronchitis requires repeated stimulations of one or two minutes each, two or three times a day. A permanent stimulation is even better here. The Chinese happily put in a surgical ligature at the appropriate points, or inject them with medications.

The Principal Points

There are two primary points to stimulate for all cases of bronchitis: the first is located on either side of the tip of the seventh cervical vertebra—the first projection beneath the nape of the neck; the second point is located two finger-widths to either side of the third thoracic vertebra—the third projection beneath the nape. For guidelines on locating these vertebral points, see page 9.

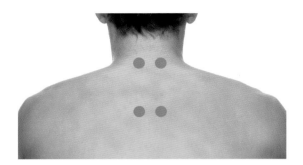
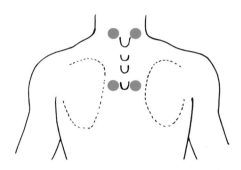

The Secondary Points

There are four secondary points—two to stimulate when treating acute bronchitis and two for the treatment of chronic bronchitis.

The first point for *acute* bronchitis is located beneath the projection of the seventh cervical vertebra; the second point is beneath the wrist crease on the lower forearm, on the spot where the radial pulse can be felt.

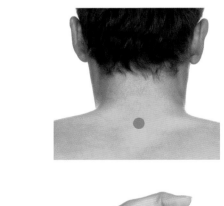
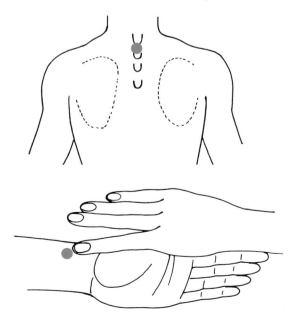

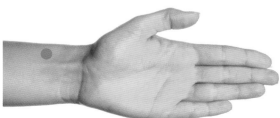

The Secondary Points (continued)

The first point for *chronic* bronchitis can be found in the notch formed where the lower bones of the index finger and thumb meet on the back of the hand.

The second point is on the outside of the calf, two finger-widths above the midpoint between the ankle and the knee.

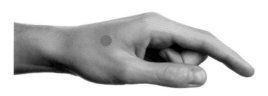

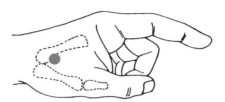

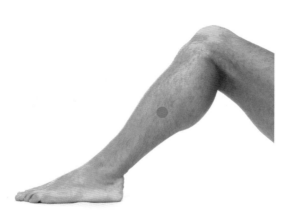

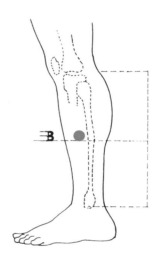

Coughs

EVERYONE HAS COUGHED or will cough. Coughing fits, barking coughs, spasmodic coughs, and whooping coughs are all familiar parts of life. But it should be clearly understood that coughing is only a symptom; it is necessary to try and trace it back to its source.

It is important to know whether a cough is productive or not—whether it is a dry cough or a wet cough that causes expectoration. As a general rule, those that are productive (carry expectorant) should not be soothed because they are serving a useful purpose. On the other hand, "dry" coughs should be given relief.

CAUSES

A complete examination of the patient is required to determine the origin of a cough. The causes are large in number, and can originate in the pulmonary system, cardiac system, nervous system, and so forth.

STANDARD TREATMENT

Basic treatment will vary quite a bit depending upon the disease responsible for causing a cough, but in general, conventional treatments will contain sedatives, the best known of which are opiate derivatives. All of these products are helpful but should not be overused because they can obstruct the elimination and expulsion of the expectorants that are burdening the bronchial tubes.

ACUPOINT TREATMENT

Whatever the cause of a cough, the stimulation of acupoints is extremely helpful: it calms coughing without obstructing expectoration, because it has no sedative properties. Once again we see the value of a "regulating" therapy like this.

TECHNIQUES TO USE

For coughing fits, vigorously massage the principal points until the coughing stops. The first point described in this chapter is one that the Chinese stimulate quite deeply. If using an electrical means of stimulation, this means the sensor has to be pressed firmly against the sternum.

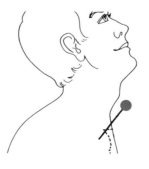

Acupuncture stimulation of the first principal point

The Principal Points

The first point is at the bottom of the throat, in a hollow above the top edge of the sternum.

The second point is a group of four points, found on the palm side of the fingers (excluding the thumb). The point is located on the joint between the first and second phalanges.

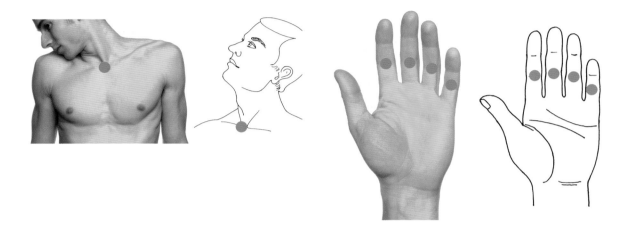

The Secondary Points

The first secondary point is on the crease of the wrist, just below the thumb; the second point is in the notch that forms where the bones of the thumb and index finger meet.

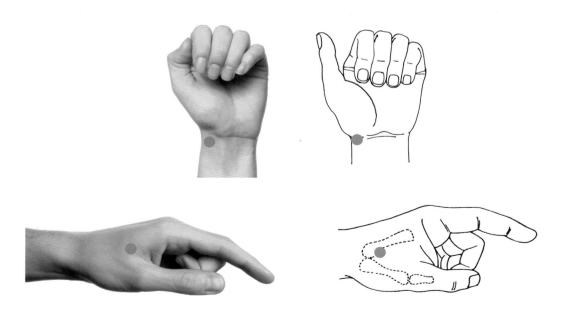

PART TEN

Nervous System

Coma

WHILE A COMA always involves a loss of consciousness, the degree of unconsciousness can vary from a light coma—from which the patient can emerge and even respond to a few questions when vigorously shaken, to a deep coma, in which the patient shows no reactions whatsoever. This unconsciousness can be so pronounced as to compromise even the most vital functions like breathing and swallowing.

In all cases coma is a very serious condition and the terminal stage of its development is often death. Therefore every possible step should be taken and all means implemented to first pull the patient back out of his torpor and then to treat the cause that led to the coma.

CAUSES

All serious illnesses can lead to coma, but some circumstances can cause a sudden coma:

- Trauma to the cranial region
- Acute cases of meningitis, especially in children
- Vascular incidents such as cerebral hemorrhaging or thrombosis—the sudden obstruction of a brain artery by a blood clot

- Comas triggered by an acute poisoning, such as would be the case for an attempted suicide, or by poisoning from within due to diabetes, urea, and so forth

STANDARD TREATMENT

There is no need for a detailed description here of the many treatments that are implemented for treating coma. These treatments are always extremely complicated and require a hospital stay to be applied.

ACUPOINT TREATMENT

The only real role for acupoint therapy is as emergency treatment while waiting for conventional treatment, but it can be considerably helpful at this juncture.

Vigorous stimulation can often cause a patient to come out of his coma. The etymology of the popular French term for undertaker, *croque-mort* (meaning "bites the dead") offers a very revealing anecdote in this regard. When there was ever any doubt whether the victim of a coma was truly dead, the undertaker would viciously bite the finger of the individual before proceeding with burial preparations. If the person was still alive, this would revive him.

As can be seen below, two of the three

sets of acupoints for the treatment of coma are indeed on the fingers.

TECHNIQUES TO USE

This is an emergency situation in which every minute counts.

It is of course vitally necessary to get the patient to the nearest hospital as soon as possible but while waiting for the ambulance or while on the way there, you can stimulate the points by whatever means you have available: massage, electrical charge, or needles with a metallic point.

The points need deep stimulation. You may even be fortunate enough to see the patient come out of his coma and reach the hospital in better condition.

The Points

There are three groups of points; the first are located on both sides at the tip of the little finger, on the skin just outside the two lower corners of the nail.

The second point is on the bottom of the feet, at the junction of the two creases created when the toes are bent forward.

Finally, the last set of points is located beneath the nails of the ten fingers, right at each fingertip.

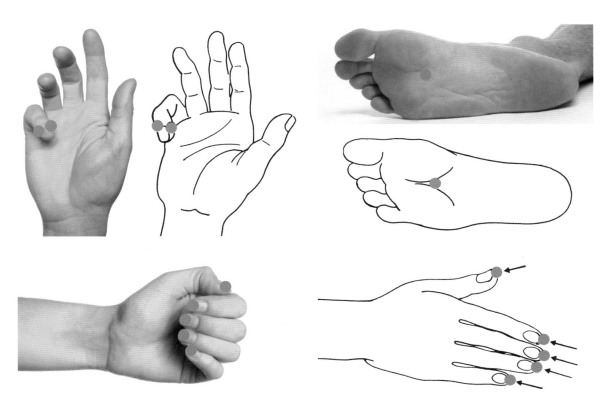

Epilepsy

IN ITS CLASSIC form, epilepsy is an abrupt loss of consciousness that causes an individual to slump or fall down. This is followed by a period of muscular spasms accompanied by symptoms of varying intensity: loss of urine, drooling, lolling of the tongue. The return to consciousness is a slow and painful process.

SYMPTOMS AND FORMS

The definition provided above is the description of the major epileptic seizure, once known as the *grand mal*—a term that has now been abandoned in favor of *tonic-clonic seizure,* which goes through three successive stages:

1. Tonic, during which the patient drops like a stone
2. Clonic, during which the patient's muscles spasm
3. Stupor, during which the patient remains confused and remembers nothing of what just happened

This is the most frequent form of this disease, but there are two others that can either exist independently, or can alternate with this seizure.

Jackson's epilepsy (or Bravais-Jackson epilepsy) is a form of the disease in which the sufferer does not lose consciousness, but witnesses a portion of his body—an arm, for example—undergo a seizure of uncontrollable spasms, which can last for a varying duration.

In the *petit mal*—whose preferred term is now *absence seizure,* as this is its most notable manifestation—the afflicted person, who is often in the midst of speaking, will abruptly stop and seem to stare off into space or at some imaginary point. After several seconds or minutes, he will resume talking or whatever he was doing, having no memory of the temporary suspension of his consciousness.

CAUSES

Epilepsies can be divided into two main categories: those for which a cause can be determined, and those for which no cause is detectable, which are known as idiopathic or "essential" epilepsies.

There are a large number of known causes for epileptic seizures: skull trauma, cerebral infections, deformity of the brain's vessels, and most importantly, brain tumors. It is because of this last risk that it is necessary to be super-vigilant when epilepsy makes its first appearance in an adult.

When a cause cannot be determined, it is considered an idiopathic form of the disease, but thanks to examination methods now available—particularly the electroencephalogram and imaging scans such as the MRI, CT, and PET scans—this second category is shrinking rapidly in proportion to the first, which is a great blessing.

Sometimes epilepsy will disappear on its own, especially among adults. Most often, however, the disease pursues a capricious course over an entire lifetime, becoming a constant threat to the patient as a seizure can occur at any time, for example when the person is on a ladder or at the steering wheel.

STANDARD TREATMENT

Outside of those cases where a curable cause can be found, conventional treatment consists mainly of prescribing chemical medications to be taken for a long time if not indefinitely. These medications play only a protective role and have no healing effects.

ACUPOINT TREATMENT

The role of acupoint therapy is quite modest when it comes to epilepsy, because it cannot replace conventional treatment. The best that can be hoped for is a stabilization of the symptoms and a reduction in the amount of medication the patient has to take.

TECHNIQUES TO USE

It is difficult to provide specific instructions here. No method yet available can stop a seizure once it has been triggered. Caregivers must be satisfied with putting the afflicted individual in a comfortable position and cushioning his or her head to help avoid injury. DO NOT place anything in the person's mouth: epileptic patients do not swallow their tongues.

On the other hand, massage of the appropriate points for several minutes in the morning and in the evening can, as I've noted elsewhere, help to reduce the quantity of medication the patient needs.

The Principal Point

The principal point is located at the base of the spine, midway between the two dimples that mark the joints of the sacrum and pelvis.

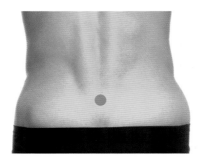
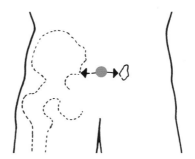

The Secondary Points

One of these points is located at the top of the skull, at the point crossed by a median line running from one ear to the other. The other point is on the edge of the occiput, right at its center.

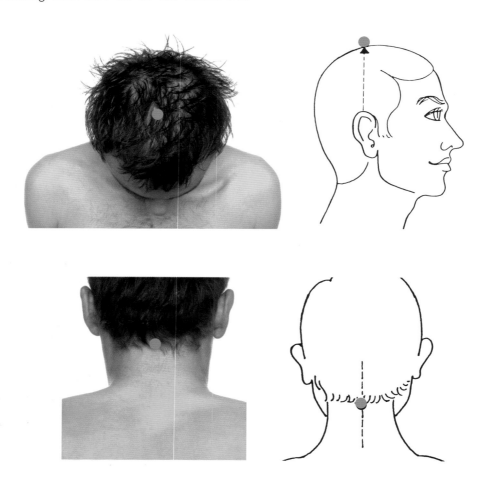

Facial Paralysis, Bell's Palsy

FACIAL MUSCLES CAN become paralyzed when the nerve that stimulates them is damaged. As each half of the face derives its motor function from a different nerve, this kind of paralysis will usually affect only one side of the face.

This one-sided affliction creates a characteristic appearance, in which the sufferer's face is twisted and pulled to one side. This will be the healthy side, because the muscles there still function and retain their tone. The ailing side of the face is flabby: the wrinkles of the skin disappear, the eye no longer closes, and the lips puff out with every breath, as if the sufferer was smoking a pipe.

Sometimes facial paralysis will affect only the forehead or mouth, but it generally affects the entire face.

CAUSES

It is important to make the distinction between the two major causes:

- Some cases of facial paralysis originate in the central nervous system or the brain. This could be due to an embolism or hemorrhage in the brain near where the root of the facial nerve is located, for example. But it is rare in these cases for the paralysis to be limited to the area of the nerve; it will more likely affect one half of the entire body, and this will be the side opposite from the stricken side of the face.

- Most often, fortunately, the nerve has only been attacked along the periphery of its course. This is the ailment known as Bell's palsy, which can be caused by a virus attacking the nerve or a small hemorrhage along its course.

STANDARD TREATMENT

While conventional medicine had little to offer this disorder for a long time, its treatment has become more and more effective. In the domain of medication, cortisone unquestionably reduces the inflammation and thus hastens recuperation. There are also surgical options in cases where manual decompression of the nerve can bring about an even faster recovery.

Finally, we should not overlook facial exercises, the physical therapy you can do yourself when standing in front of a mirror. This works just as effectively on the small muscles as it does on the big ones.

ACUPOINT TREATMENT

Acupuncture and acupressure stand among the best treatments for facial paralysis. It has allowed brilliant, rapid, and incident-free recoveries to take place.

Treatment requires repeated sessions and generally vigorous styles of stimulation—such as electrical stimulation or needle acupuncture—combined with frequent sessions of self-massage (every two hours, for example). Though this is a demanding treatment, it is well worth it for the speedy recovery it engenders.

TECHNIQUES TO USE

The points should be stimulated as soon as possible after the symptoms develop. It is a good idea to turn to vigorous methods of stimulation, especially electric acupuncture, but it is vital that the patient also take an active role in his treatment by stimulating the points himself several times a day.

Even when the disease is old and complicated by after-effects, acupoint therapy can still offer hope of a strong recovery and the restoration of the face to nearly its normal appearance. Therapy can be beneficially combined with facial physical therapy.

The Principal Points

The first principal point is on the palm side of the wrist, approximately three finger-widths beneath the crease; the exact spot is where the radial pulse can be felt. The second point is on the back edge of the skull, three finger-widths in from the ears on either side.

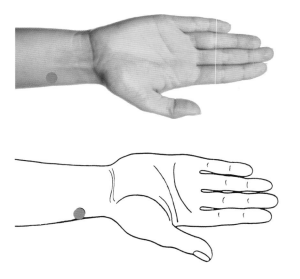
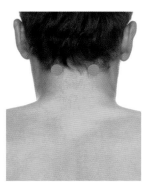
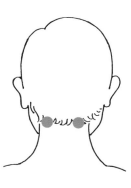

The Secondary Points

These points can be found around each affected area. For treating the forehead, use the point two finger-widths above the center of the eyebrow; for the cheek, stimulate the point on the inner edge of the orbit of the eye; for the chin, the point is two finger-widths on either side of the center of the chin.

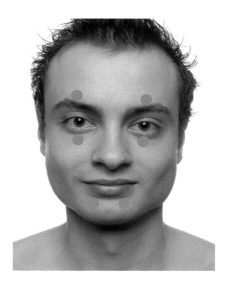

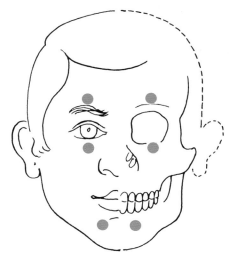

Other Forms of Paralysis

WHEN MOTOR NERVE function is interrupted, paralysis ensues in one or more parts of the body. Its origin can lie in an attack anywhere along the course of a nerve—from the brain, where specialized zones can be found that correspond with various parts of the body, down to the ends of the nerve filaments.

An accurate description of the many diseases that can involve some type of paralysis could run to several medical tomes. I am therefore going to be satisfied with simply describing their formal principles; in any case, our therapy depends more upon the area that has been affected than on the original cause.

FORMS AND CAUSES

In the infinite variety of nerve afflictions, we can still find several broad outlines.

- Hemiplegia describes paralysis of one side of the body, either the right or the left side. This condition is generally caused by a disorder affecting a brain artery, such as bleeding from a cerebral hemorrhage or obstruction from a thrombosis.
- Paraplegia refers to paralysis of the lower half of the body and its two lower limbs. Spinal cord damage—often from an accident—is the most common cause of this disorder. Because the spine has been cut, the lower limbs and lower body organs are no longer able to function. Therefore paraplegia is often accompanied by troubles emptying the bladder or intestines.
- Multiple paralyses can affect different regions of the body, such as a hand and a leg, for example. The quintessential cause of this kind of condition is multiple sclerosis, a disorder that destroys the brain and spinal cord with plaques or lesions in different areas that thereby create scattered and varied forms of paralysis. The plaques are characterized by destruction of the myelin sheath that surrounds each neuron and speeds the transmission of signals throughout the central nervous system.

STANDARD TREATMENT

It must be recognized that we are cruelly at a loss when confronted by the different forms of paralysis. Some are permanent, while others do respond to treatment. In all cases, recovery of the nervous system is slow and difficult, requiring patience and stubborn courage. Physical therapy is the best treatment, with regular sessions and relentless work.

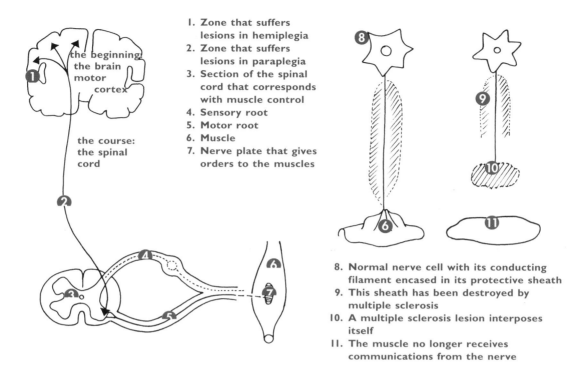

1. Zone that suffers lesions in hemiplegia
2. Zone that suffers lesions in paraplegia
3. Section of the spinal cord that corresponds with muscle control
4. Sensory root
5. Motor root
6. Muscle
7. Nerve plate that gives orders to the muscles

8. Normal nerve cell with its conducting filament encased in its protective sheath
9. This sheath has been destroyed by multiple sclerosis
10. A multiple sclerosis lesion interposes itself
11. The muscle no longer receives communications from the nerve

The motor function path

Medications are systematically tried—especially the vitamins B₁, B₁₂, and so on—without any real certainty about their effect. Some small hopes have been aroused with the discovery of substances capable of inspiring nerve growth, but they are still in the middle of what will be a long experimental stage.

In similar fashion, surgery is now audaciously embarking on operations to implant batteries that deliver electrical stimulation to paralyzed nerves.

ACUPOINT TREATMENT

Acupoint therapy should be combined with other treatments as described above, because it helps and reinforces them. But these, too, have to be practiced diligently and regularly, with energy and tenacity.

TECHNIQUES TO USE

Always choose a point at the root along with one or two points from the lesion area that will change at every session (see below).

Also combine continuous stimulation methods such as electrical acupuncture with manual massages. These should take place for two minutes, two or three times a day. This sounds onerous, but a clear improvement will gradually take place, rewarding the patient's efforts and those of the people around him.

The Points

All of these points are equal in importance; they can be divided into two categories—points at the roots and points at the lesions.

Points at the roots: In cases of hemiplegia, these points are located on the head, with the most important being the one at the top of the skull, at the point crossed by a median line running from one ear to the other. Another point is located in the center of the neck, against the edge of the skull at the hairline. For paraplegia, the root point to stimulate is located in the lumbar region above the sacrum, beneath the last vertebra that can be felt by the finger (fourth lumbar vertebra).

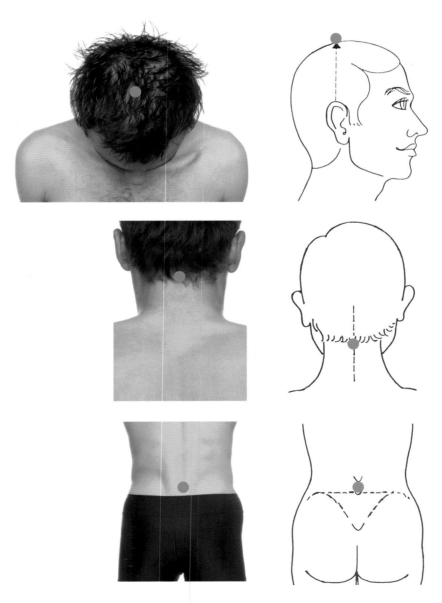

Points at the lesions: For the *shoulder*, use the point at the middle of its slope; for the *arm*, at the outside end of the elbow crease; for the *forearm*, the point is in the middle of that limb (on the top side, halfway between wrist and elbow, and halfway between the two sides); for the *hand*, in the center of the back of the hand; for the *fingers*, on the back of the hand, in the middle of the second joint of each finger.

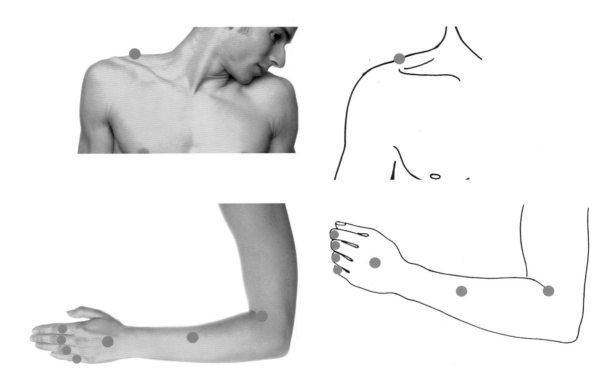

The Points (continued)

For the *hip*, the point is just behind the head of the femur; for the *thigh*, in the center of the front and back surfaces; for the *foot*, in the center of the dorsal crease of the foot; for the *toes*, at the base of each one; for the *leg*, just in front of the head of the fibula.

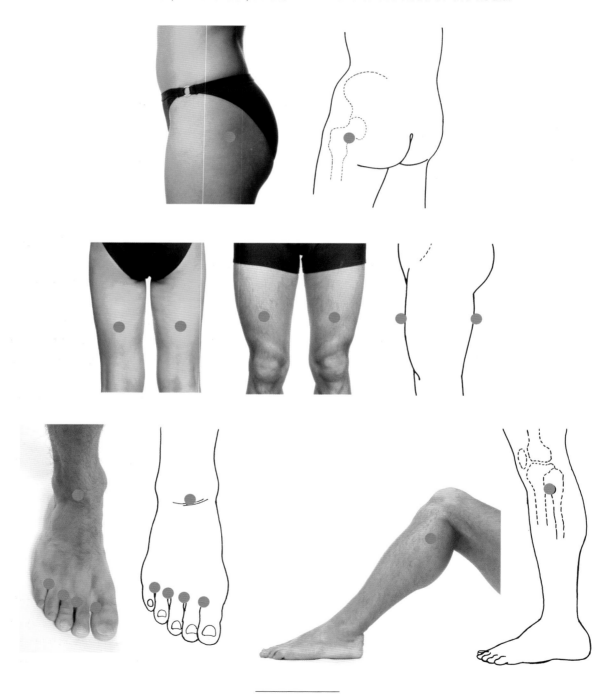

Intoxicants:
Drugs, Alcohol, and Tobacco

FOR MILLENNIA, MANKIND has sought out substances that can be used to alter the mind and behavior through stimulation or sedation. In addition to the most common intoxicants—alcohol and tobacco—there are many different kinds of drugs available.

Because there are so many different kinds of drugs, they have a number of different effects. It is customary to divide them into "soft drugs" and "hard drugs"—the chief representatives of the first category being marijuana and hashish, and those of the second category opium derivatives such as heroin. Hallucinogens like LSD are often put in their own category, as are prescription drugs. However, "druggie" researchers seem to be adept at harnessing the most recent discoveries of modern chemistry for their own purposes, and new drugs are constantly appearing on the scene.

SYMPTOMS

Symptoms of hard drug use can be difficult to identify. Be wary of any bizarre behavior that includes wild mood swings ranging from aggressiveness to excessive angelic innocence. Users may resort to criminal behavior to support their drug use, and they can contract infections such as, hepatitis, AIDS, and blood poisoning from dirty needles. In addition, emergencies like accidents and overdoses are always possible, ending up with the death of the user—all too often an adolescent whose corpse will be discovered in some sleazy dump.

However, the manifestations of alcohol are hardly a mystery to anyone. Acute alcohol intoxication is first marked by a phase of euphoric excitation that develops into incoherent language and clumsy movements. Further drinking will cause the drinker to collapse into a heavy sleep, perhaps after vomiting. The subject is dead drunk at this point, and in some cases might be just plain dead. Generally, however, the individual will come to in a few hours with a severe headache and nausea, all the classic symptoms of a hangover. If this goes no further and the individual does not relapse, it will have no long-lasting harmful consequences.

The same cannot be said about chronic alcoholism, in which a person becomes dependent on alcohol and continues to consume it despite adverse physical, mental, and social consequences. The main physical symptoms of long-term alcohol abuse are digestive and nerve-related. Digestive disorders begin with an irritation of the mouth, esophagus, and stomach, followed by heartburn and acidic vomiting. These can lead to the development of severe pancreas and liver disease, eventually creating cirrhosis. Nerve disorders related to alcoholism will affect the lower limbs and can even create a partial paralysis of the legs. But they also affect the brain, causing behavioral disorders that can lead to imbecility and dementia, with all the family and social disasters this entails.

We then come to tobacco last, but it is certainly not least! True, it has only been a relatively short time since we realized that smoking—long considered a pleasant and life-enhancing pastime—is terribly harmful. Yet tobacco use increases the two scourges of the modern world: circulatory diseases and cancer.

CAUSES

Why do people take drugs, drink, and/or smoke? It seems that there are elements these intoxicants have in common, and other elements that are specific to each one.

Drug use, at least among the young, is a relatively new phenomenon in the West. It can be fueled by escapism or a rejection of society, or even just a desire to be "cool." All these elements seem to play an equal role.

Alcoholism has long been a constant in our societies; our civilization could even be described as bathing in alcohol. But not everyone becomes an alcoholic. A distinction should be made between the excessive drinker—the individual who can stop when-

ever he wishes—and the true alcoholic, who is truly an addict.

Lastly, there are two common motivations for tobacco use: One is individual—smoking is equivalent to breastfeeding as the sucking reflex (the first reflex movement made by the newborn child) is the preeminent soothing reflex. The other is social—smoking with other people is taking part in a ritual in which the ancestral symbol of fire plays an essential role.

STANDARD TREATMENT

Any efforts at addressing intoxicant addiction require strong psychological and social support: organizations like rehab centers, support groups, alcoholics anonymous, and so on are vitally important for the addict looking to make a change. But new medications and methods now available also offer a valuable contribution to these efforts.

For example, medications like naloxone or some anti-hypertensives are now used successfully to treat hard drug users. Sulfured medications like disulfiram that block the action of alcohol on the liver are now used to treat alcoholism. While no specific anti-intoxicant has yet been found to counter tobacco, nicotine-containing gums and patches can sometimes help people break the habit of smoking.

ACUPOINT TREATMENT

Since the British first brought opium to China, the Chinese have been dealing with drug problems. For this reason they have well-established and effective treatment programs.

Alcohol and tobacco, on the contrary, offer new territory for acupuncture. Research looking for effective treatment methods is ongoing in this field, but acupoint therapy already seems to be enjoying substantial success.

TECHNIQUES TO USE

Research shows that manual stimulation for fifteen minutes or electrical stimulation for ten minutes—once in the morning and once in the evening for either method—are effective treatments.

The Principal Point

One point is common for all the ill effects caused by intoxicants. It is located on the lateral side of the head, a hand-width above the auricle of the ear.

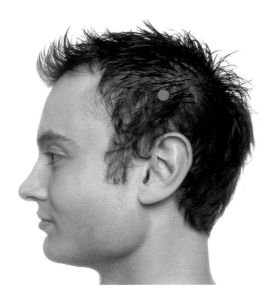
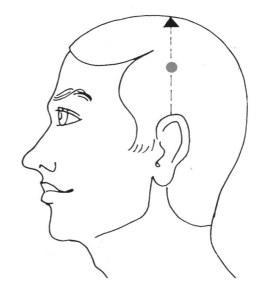

The Secondary Points

For *drug abuse*, a study performed in Toulouse, France, has demonstrated the value of stimulating two points, preferably with electricity. One of the points is on the back edge of the skull at the hairline, two finger-widths from the ear; the other is on the bridge of the nose.

For *alcohol*, the point is at the end of the nose. For *tobacco*, stimulate the entire zone encompassing the root of the helix on the ear.

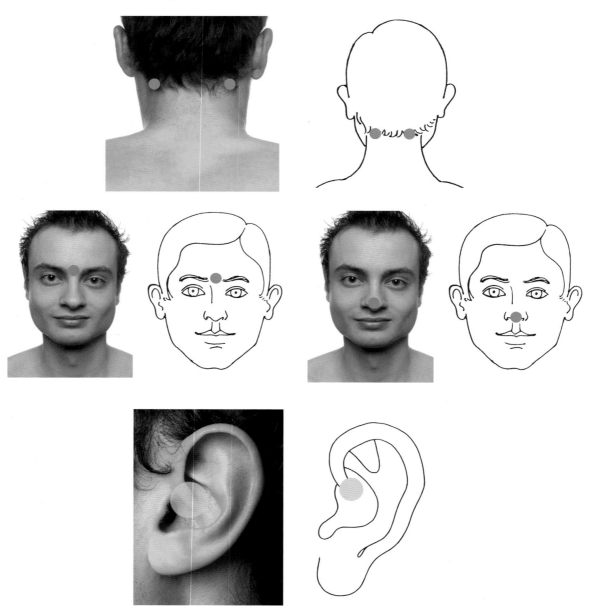

Depression

THERE IS NO disorder that is as difficult to define or establish boundaries of as *depression*—a blanket term for all those mental states in which the individual no longer feels good about herself, is ill at ease and dissatisfied with life, and even feels alienated from herself.

The patient depreciates her own worth and feels she is useless and incapable of doing anything well. In the end these become self-fulfilling prophecies. She wallows in anxiety and the slightest incident is more than she can handle. The emotional symptoms can be accompanied by physical ones, such as a tendency to shiver. Insomnia is commonly present.

In truth, depression has been called various things across the ages: neurasthenia, spleen, cerebral anemia, and in modern times simply depression. For some, the pain of it is felt all the more intensely because of the way it eludes definition.

CAUSES

A depressed person will sometimes attribute her illness to specific causes—life's hardships and the routine drudgery that characterizes most lives. A life that feels compartmentalized into commuting, working, and sleeping drains a person's enthusiasm and interest and strips away all courage. This is how this disease is actually quite typical of its time and its society.

However, it seems that current discoveries have identified many physiological factors involved in the disorder. It can often be a hereditary condition exacerbated by blood disorders like tetany or spasmophilia, caused by a decrease in the body's levels of calcium or magnesium. Neurotransmitters like serotonin are also clearly involved in many cases of depression.

STANDARD TREATMENT

For a long time, depression was treated with tranquilizers. And it is true that with this kind of medication we were able to alter a mental state for the first time. But success has gone far beyond what was hoped for, so to speak. Tranquillizers are now the most commonly used medications in the world; their sales can be measured in tons. Unfortunately, they are not devoid of drawbacks, among which are the encouragement of somnolence and apathy. Furthermore, because resistance to them has increased, the doses needed to be effective have also increased, thus creating a dangerous therapeutic escalation.

In recent years, new classes of

anti-depressant medications have helped millions of people. Tricyclic anti-depressants, MAO inhibitors, and SSRIs (selective serotonin re-uptake inhibitors), as well as other atypical medications all have significant success rates in the treatment of depression. They don't work for everyone however, and often have difficult side effects.

ACUPOINT TREATMENT

For the above reasons, it is therefore valuable to have a method that is safe and can bring help to people suffering from depression.

Acupoint therapy can be combined with any other treatment and should gradually lead to the partial or even complete reduction of medications.

TECHNIQUES TO USE

With depression, we do not massage points so much as we massage entire zones. Because depression is a chronic ailment, it is helpful to stimulate the points and zones several times every day, for several minutes at a time.

Note: When the patient is prey to an acute anxiety attack, there is one point that should be stimulated immediately. It is located on the front of the chest four finger-widths beneath the clavicle on the right side. (For illustrations of this point location, see Stage Fright, page 265.)

The Points

The first zone for treating depression is along the crease of the wrist.

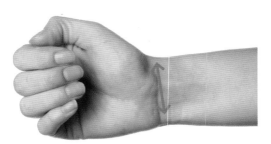
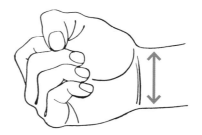

The second zone is on the abdomen—it is the median line running between the sternum and the navel. The third point (and the zone around it) is located on the very top of the head at the intersection of the median line with a line going from one ear to the other.

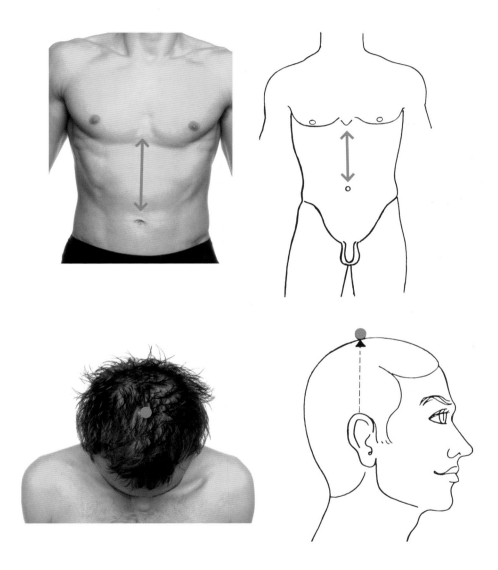

Schizophrenia, Psychosis, and Other Serious Mental Disorders

IT WAS ONCE standard to divide the profusion of mental diseases into two categories: neuroses and psychoses. This determination was based on the notion that neurotics, whatever kind of problems they might have, are generally able to maintain contact with reality. For example, the subject could be experiencing hallucinations but still recognize them as being external phenomena. Psychotics, on the contrary, experience everything as a part of themselves and cannot tell the difference between their inner world and the world outside. The psychotic was traditionally the one diagnosed as insane.

However, modern research and therapies have recognized that neurotics exist who have mental confusion, and that some psychotics can achieve self-identification and lead normal lives with treatment.

SYMPTOMS AND FORMS

There are several different types of psychosis; below I will discuss the three most prevalent.

- Schizophrenia is the most serious disorder, first and foremost because it strikes the young—typical onset occurs between fifteen and thirty-five years old. It is believed that 1 percent of everyone this age is afflicted. Its onset can be sudden, with the appearance of delirium and abnormal actions, or gradual, characterized by bizarre behavior, laughing for no reason, total immobility, or dangerous aggressive acts. If left untreated, schizophrenia will lead eventually to complete personality dissolution and true madness.

- Bipolar disorder, formerly called manic-depressive psychosis, is characterized by mood swings between depressive states during which the subject, in the depths of despondency, is filled with thoughts of self-hatred and recrimination and accuses himself of every sin and crime. Suicide is a real danger at these times. On the other side of this mood pendulum are manic states during which the subject is in a state of euphoria and can even appear intoxicated. Sometimes the alternations between these states take several months, sometimes only days.

- Delusional disorder is characterized by external delirium. The patient believes things that are not generally recognized as true—that people are eavesdropping on him, for example, or persecuting or threatening him. People suffering from this kind of paranoid delusions have even been known to file charges in court or complain to the police about their family and neighbors.

In addition to these standard forms, there are many cases of mental disease that are hard to classify but are generally comparable in some respects to these three main categories.

CAUSES

Ideas about mental disease have, like everything else, evolved in accordance with their times.

Following a period in which everything was thought to have a physiological origin and doctors hunted for lesions in specific zones of the brain, the medical establishment began to believe that mental illness was a purely psychological disorder, linked to the individual's emotions and social environment. Today we have come full circle and are back to focusing on physiological causes. This has been inspired by recent discoveries concerning disorders in brain cell function. As always, every era provides its own portion of the truth.

Sometimes, although it is fairly rare, anatomical lesions (tumors, for example),

can cause psychosis. Environment also has a huge role to play, and while it may not be the ultimate determining factor, a family that offers the patient secure and reassuring surroundings is the best indication for the healing of a mental disease.

But the greatest progress has been made possible by the study of brain chemistry, especially the study of the famous neuropeptides that transmit impulses from one brain cell to another. For instance, there is some evidence to suggest that schizophrenia is linked with defective processing of endorphin, a potent neuropeptide. This is only the beginning of an arduous but promising course of research.

STANDARD TREATMENT

Mental disease treatments were turned upside down with the appearance of pharmaceutical therapy. Before the 1980s, hardly anything but electroshock treatments and a handful of anti-psychotic medications offered any improvement. Nowadays, treatment has largely given way to chemical medications, essentially neuroleptics and tranquillizers. Lithium, which is a metal, should be singled out for its quasi-specific effect on one disorder in particular: bipolar disorder.

ACUPOINT TREATMENT

If, at first glance, there are any diseases that appear well beyond the reach of acupoint therapy, it would be mental disease. And yet in China, there are entire psychiatric hospitals dedicated to the treatment of schizophrenia using traditional Chinese medicine.

TECHNIQUES TO USE

There can be no question—let me make this quite clear from the start—of undertaking this kind of treatment at home. I am only citing it here to show the kind of results acupoint therapy can provide when properly and systematically applied.

In Chinese hospitals, schizophrenics receive sessions of electric acupuncture every day, using some of the points described in this chapter. Chinese exercises and poetry-writing are also part of the standard treatment regimen; they help the patient to open up and get back in touch with himself physically and mentally. The results of this kind of treatment are comparable with those provided by pharmaceutical based treatments. How sad it is that we don't have health centers like this here!

The Principal Points

The first point is at the very top of the head (at the tallest point of the body), at the junction of the median line and the line passing over the top of the auricles of both ears.

The second principal point is above the upper lip, at the point two-thirds down from the nose and one third up from the top of the lip.

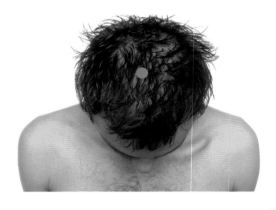

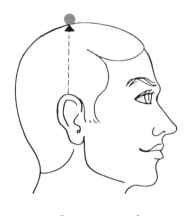

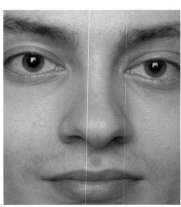

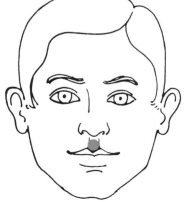

The Secondary Points

The first secondary point is located on the bridge of the nose between the eyebrows.
The second is at the bottom of the sternum.

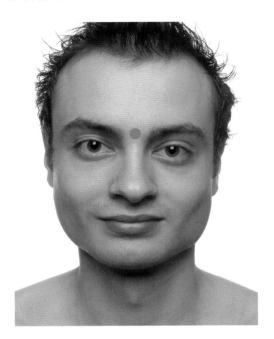

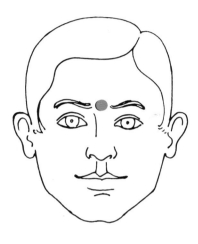

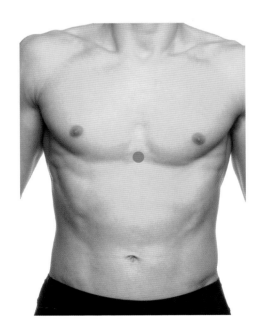

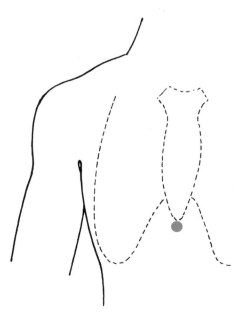

PART ELEVEN

Reproductive Health

Impotence

IMPOTENCE IS A blanket term that describes a man's inability to have normal sexual relations. It occurs in three main forms:

- The subject feels no sexual desire.
- The penis remains soft and cannot achieve penetration. This is an erectile dysfunction.
- The individual "comes" too quickly. This is premature ejaculation, which can prevent the individual from having a satisfying relationship.

CAUSES

It is tempting to lay the blame for impotence on a disorder of male hormones. This is actually rarely the case. Impotence is often psychological in origin. This is almost always true for cases involving the lack of desire or premature ejaculation, but—and this is a new discovery—it is less often implicated in erectile dysfunction.

With erectile dysfunction, it has been found that the cause is more often due to a problem with the vessels that carry blood to the penis. This is because the ability to get an erection depends upon the blood vessels, especially the arteries. At a specific moment they dilate and fill the organ with blood. If the vessels are impaired in any way, or even more so if they are clogged, then the entire process will be obstructed.

STANDARD TREATMENT

Viagra and related medications have become the most common treatment by far for erectile dysfunction. In cases where it does not help, some surgical treatments do exist for clearing and/or replacing the arteries. For other impotence issues, there are less common interventions such as psychological counseling and even prosthetic penises. All of this "play" in physical and psychological domains requires experienced practitioners, and the last decade has witnessed the genesis of an entire new body of medical specialists: sexologists. They need to be able to deal with the psychology of individuals and couples as deftly as they apply surgical instruments.

This is because a man's sex life, and the reproductive function associated with it, touches on the deepest levels of his personality. After all, this provided Freud the building blocks for his notion of mental life. Many centuries before Freud, the Chinese regarded sexual energy as one of the primary sources for vital energy.

ACUPOINT TREATMENT

Because the Chinese have confronted issues of sexual vitality for millennia, they have studied it most diligently and have isolated some successful treatments for it. Of course, in territory that shifts as much as this one, no results can be guaranteed. But the innocuous nature and simplicity of the method makes it a tool of choice. Perseverance is called for here; acupoint treatment can also, as elsewhere, be combined with any other therapy.

TECHNIQUES TO USE

The best results seem to come from stimulating the points one after the other with moderate pressure for five to fifteen minutes, morning and night. This can be done manually, with a needle, or with electricity, and should be performed for ten days in a row.

A week's break should be taken before resuming for the same period of time outlined above, followed by another rest period, and so on.

The Chinese also inject vitamins or male hormones into these points.

The Principal Points

The first principal point is located on the lower back. It is on the lumbar spine on a level with the top of the iliac crests.

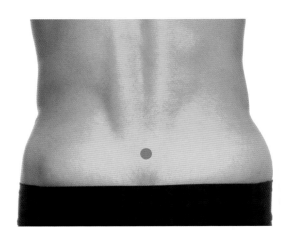

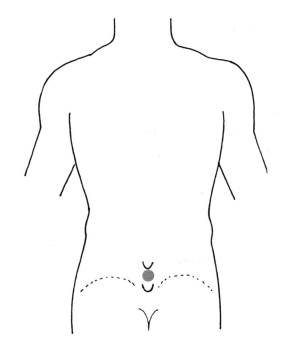

The Principal Points (continued)

The second point is located on the inside of the lower calf, a hand-width above the ankle bone in a small notch along the back edge of the tibia.

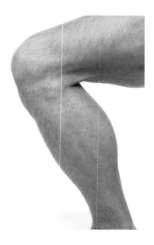
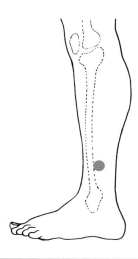

The Secondary Points

The first secondary point is located on the abdomen halfway between the navel and the pubic bone. The second point is at the end of the wrist crease beneath the little finger.

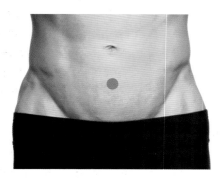
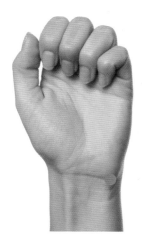
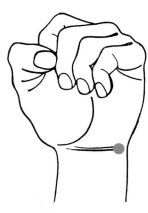
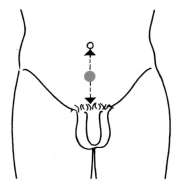

Prostate Disease

THE PROSTATE IS located beneath the bladder, which rests on top of it like a lamp on its pedestal. The upper part of the urethra canal crosses through the prostate carrying urine from the bladder to outside the body. The prostate is considered a secondary genital gland because it creates a fluid that nourishes the sperm. However, its intricate fit inside the urinary apparatus makes it a prime target of all the health problems that can afflict the urinary system.

SYMPTOMS AND FORMS

Knowing this, we can easily grasp why the pathological conditions of the prostate are

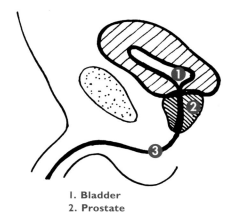

1. Bladder
2. Prostate
3. Urethra

Normal prostate

revealed primarily by urinary symptoms. These conditions include the common problems of prostatitis, adenoma (BPH), and cancer.

Prostatitis is an inflammation of the prostate. It may be linked to a bacterial infection, or may have no identifiable cause. The bacteria responsible for it can come from the urinary tract or even from a more distant infection like boils or pulmonary tuberculosis. The disease usually starts suddenly with shivering, high fever, and pain in the lower belly. If no treatment is undertaken it can quickly form an abscess that will open on to the urethra or contaminate a testicle. Vigorous treatment will generally cure the abscess and its consequences. But if this does not work, the disease will develop into chronic prostatitis with periods of calm and periodic "flare-ups."

Benign prostatic hypertrophy (BPH), the prostate problem most common in elderly men, is much more frequent. It refers to the enlargement and partial hardening of the prostate gland. Unfortunately, this enlargement can interfere with the body's ability to void urine.

The presence of prostate cancer, meanwhile, is revealed by a series of symptoms similar to those caused by BPH but their development is much more rapid. It can also be part of a metastasis from a cancer that has spread from other organs. However, prostate cancer is fairly easy to sniff out, and responds very well to early treatment. It is one of the rare cancers that has a biological "signature," in this case a rise in the rate of certain chemical markers in the blood, the best known of which is acid phosphatase.

CAUSES

We have seen that prostatitis can be due to an infection of the gland by a variety of germs (coli bacillus, staphylococcus, and even the bacillus of tuberculosis).

The causes of BPH are unknown; all that can be said is that this disease is a little like uterine fibroids in women, but modern medicine is still forced to confess its ignorance concerning all the rest.

Alas, the same is true about prostate cancer! All that we know is that it is often very dependent upon hormones, aggravated by male hormones and improved, on the contrary, by female hormones.

STANDARD TREATMENT

Bacterial prostatitis requires intense antibiotic treatment as early as possible to prevent its development into a chronic condition.

BPH sometimes receives no treatment at all: some men can live with it until the end of their lives, experiencing very little discomfort. There are often flare-ups after an exhausting situation (a long car ride, for example) but everything can be quickly restored to order with some herbal medicine—the most common of which is saw palmetto berry. There are a few different classes of medications to treat the disease if necessary, and as a last resort, surgeries.

Prostate cancer may be treated with female hormones, or the more specialized male anti-hormones. In addition, radiation or surgery may be required.

ACUPOINT TREATMENT

Acupoint therapy can only play a supporting role in the case of prostatitis and cancer, but it is can be a major component in treatment of BPH. The therapy can calm flare-ups, halt spasms, and reestablish a more normal urine flow.

TECHNIQUES TO USE

A urine retention crisis requires very strong stimulation—by hand or electrically—until it has been resolved. Chronic prostate symptoms do not require such strong stimulation, but they do benefit from longer stimulation: twenty minutes both morning and evening.

The Principal Points

The first point is located on the lower back, three finger-widths away from the lumbar spine on a line even with the tops of the iliac crests; the second point can be found three finger-widths away on either side of the anus.

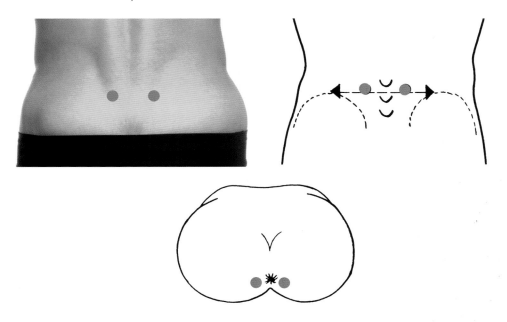

The Secondary Points

The first secondary point is located on the lower abdomen halfway between the navel and the pubic bone; the second point is located on either side of the pubic bone, on a little bony tip known as the pubic spine.

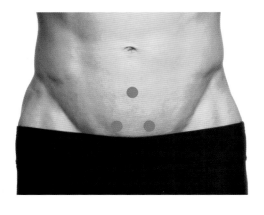

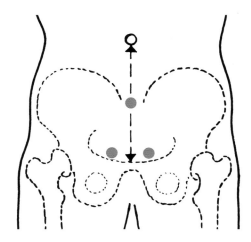

Breast Disease

THE GLAND OF lactation responsible for feeding the tiniest human beings, the breast is the very symbol of femininity and considered women's most beautiful adornment; unfortunately, this second function has almost eliminated the first in our modern societies. However, breastfeeding is making a return in the modern world, which is a good thing for both baby and mother.

SYMPTOMS AND FORMS

Almost all women feel tension in the breasts just before their period. This can be almost intolerable sometimes and can also be accompanied by an excessive increase in their size. While this is not a dangerous medical symptom, it can cause enough discomfort to be a serious problem for some women.

The conditions that should be heeded with great wariness include discharge from the nipples, a lump in the breast, and repeated scabs on the nipple area. All of these conditions require a serious medical examination.

More than 80 percent of breast lumps are benign, whether they occur singly or in several spots in the breasts. Nevertheless, once a lump has been found, it is best to have it examined by whatever methods the doctor feels will provide the best diagnosis.

Mammograms and biopsies are two of the primary options. Thermography—a method of taking detailed temperature readings of the breast to evaluate blood flow—is an increasingly common diagnostic tool that is also exceptionally safe.

But contrary to all these serious conditions, the breasts can cause problems without any actual disease being present. Many women experience breast pain that seems to have no evident cause. Still others experience pain from numerous (benign) fibrocystic lumps.

CAUSES

The breasts respond to a woman's complex gynecological balance and are therefore subject to the before- and after-effects of the menstrual cycle. It may be that imbalances in the interplay of the body's many hormones are responsible for all the benign and serious illnesses affecting the breasts, including changes in their shape or size.

Cancer is always to be dreaded as a possible cause for what may prove to be totally benign symptoms; appropriate examinations are necessary with any unusual breast symptoms that do not resolve themselves after the menstrual period.

STANDARD TREATMENT

Benign tumors like fibroids, as well as some of the cyclical disorders, can be treated effectively with hormones, but these can be difficult to administer properly.

If breast cancer is diagnosed, conventional medicine offers treatments based on chemotherapy, radiation, surgery, and so forth.

ACUPOINT TREATMENT

There is no question of using acupuncture or acupressure as the sole recourse against serious breast diseases, cancer particularly. However, benign disorders of the breast can often be helped with stimulation of the points.

In addition, these points are extremely effective for cyclical disorders and for countering any deformities of the breasts these can cause. There, as elsewhere, their use reveals the "regulatory" role of acupoint therapy, which synchronizes organ function.

TECHNIQUES TO USE

The techniques will differ depending upon the condition to be treated.

For benign tumors, the points should be stimulated several times a day for two or three minutes each time. Or a technique such as a ligature can be used to provide continuous stimulation.

For cyclical disorders, on the other hand, like swollen breasts before a period, it should be sufficient to stimulate the points eight days before the time of the next period, for ten to fifteen minutes twice a day.

The Principal Points

The first point is located on the front of the thigh, a hand-width above the kneecap's outer corner; the second point is on the inner edge of the forearm, about three finger-widths from the crease of the elbow.

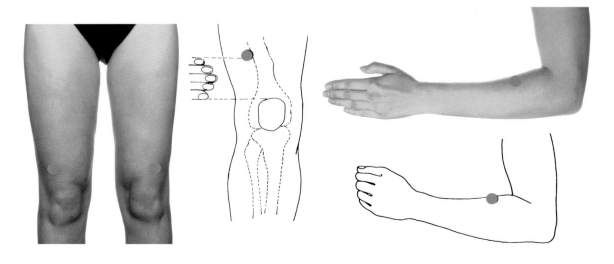

The Secondary Points

The first secondary point is on the sternum bone between the breasts, at the level of the nipples; the second point is just below each breast, about two finger-widths beneath the nipple.

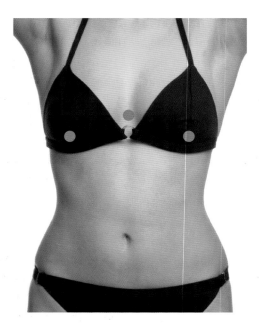

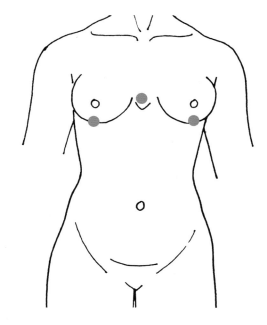

Morning Sickness

MORNING SICKNESS IS the blanket term for the feelings of nausea and vomiting that affect many women during the course of their pregnancies, especially in the first trimester.

The episodes of nausea, sometimes accompanied by actual vomiting, are so frequently associated with early pregnancy that they can be easily described as part of its initial symptoms. Sometimes a woman will only discover she is pregnant because of these symptoms.

As the popular name implies, this is most commonly a "morning" sickness. The future mother feels dizzy and queasy when she gets up, and uncustomarily ill at ease. She often starts feeling much better as the day wears on. In any event, these symptoms eventually disappear, most often after the third month of pregnancy.

But there are times when things grow worse: when the woman continues to vomit over the entire nine months, or when this vomiting, because of its frequency and size, imperils the woman's health. This is what is known as *hyperemesis gravidarum*.

CAUSES

The exact cause of morning sickness is unclear. Some theories suggest that fluctuating hormone levels are responsible, while others target the changing chemical composition of stomach and intestinal fluids. The condition does seem partially hereditary, and also vulnerable to low blood-sugar levels. Lastly, some practitioners believe that morning sickness has primarily emotional causes, and recommend psychological counseling.

STANDARD TREATMENT

Powerful anti-vomiting drugs now exist. They do not always solve the problem completely, however, and some women may need to be hospitalized to prevent dehydration.

ACUPOINT TREATMENT

Acupoint therapy is useful in the treatment of all vomiting disorders, including serious cases and those associated with pregnancy. But it is especially valuable in the more moderate cases, allowing pregnant women to dispense with the chemical drugs.

TECHNIQUES TO USE

For a woman displaying the standard symptoms, it is a good idea to stimulate the points for five or six minutes before rising in the morning. Be prepared to do a repeat session a half-hour later if the ill feelings have not passed.

In the more serious disorders, the stimulations should be repeated several times a day, and it is not out of the question to employ a form of continuous stimulation like electrical current.

The Points

The first point is located on the middle of the abdomen, at the midway point between the navel and the sternum. The second point is just next to the tip of the sternum, against the edge of the ribs. The third point is on the palm side of the wrist, roughly in the center and three finger-widths below the crease.

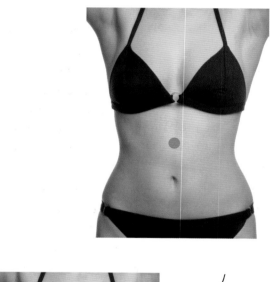

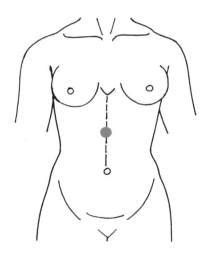

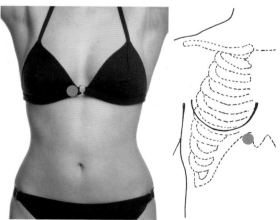

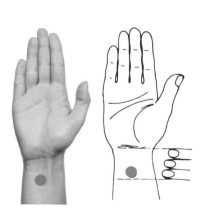

Amenorrhea:
The Absence of Menstrual Periods

AMENORRHEA IS THE clinical name for the absence of menstrual periods. It can occur in a woman who has never had a period (this is known as primary amenorrhea), or in a woman whose periods stopped after some number of normal menstrual cycles (secondary amenorrhea).

Other signs and symptoms can be associated with amenorrhea, and these should be carefully noted. They may include stomach pains and digestive symptoms like nausea and vomiting, for example, or circulatory symptoms like facial flushing and hot flashes.

CAUSES

Some causes of amenorrhea are completely natural: pregnancy is the prime example and should always be the first likely cause to be considered.

During extreme periods of women's genital life like puberty and menopause, there can be times when menstruation is halted. It is generally accepted in modern societies that the first menstruation typically begins between ten and fourteen years of age, and that menopause typically takes place between forty-five and sixty. But there can be early or late puberties and early or late cases of menopause that are completely normal.

When the absence of periods is truly abnormal, the condition can originate in a variety of ways. As can be seen in the diagram on page 246, three principal organs have a role to play in menstruation. First is the uterus, or womb, from which the blood comes and which houses the fertilized egg if there is one. Then there are the ovaries, glands that produce an egg once a month but which also, by means of the hormones they pour into the bloodstream, enable the womb to manufacture the "nest" where the fertilized egg will be housed, if fertilization takes place. If fertilization does not occur, the "nest" no longer has any purpose and will be eliminated with the blood at the end of a month's time to make way for a new cycle. But this is not the whole story. Another gland—the pituitary at the base of the brain—controls ovary function.

Causes of amenorrhea can thus originate in any of these three organs. Uterine causes can be a result of poor organ anatomy or an inability to properly utilize the hormones sent to it by the ovaries. Ovarian conditions such as cysts, failure to ovulate, or hormone dysfunctions can likewise prevent menstruation from occurring. Finally, the pituitary

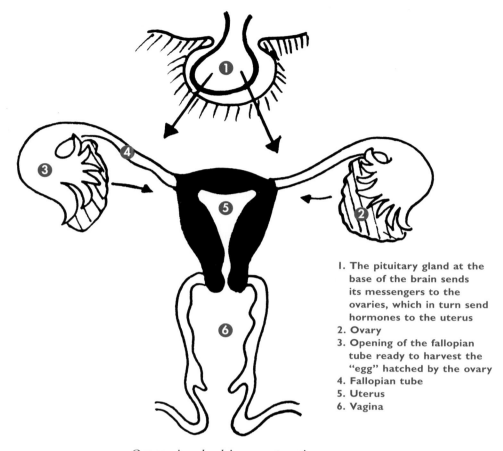

1. The pituitary gland at the base of the brain sends its messengers to the ovaries, which in turn send hormones to the uterus
2. Ovary
3. Opening of the fallopian tube ready to harvest the "egg" hatched by the ovary
4. Fallopian tube
5. Uterus
6. Vagina

Organs involved in menstruation

can be imbalanced by tumors, functional disorders, and even emotional disturbances. It is fairly common knowledge that strong emotion can stop a period . . . or start one.

For this reason, while all cases of amenorrhea require extensive examination, most of them can be traced to functional disorders rather than physiological ones—more a question of a simple breakdown than any real damage.

STANDARD TREATMENT

A certain number of cysts, tumors, and malformations are the province of the surgeon. But in many cases, hormone therapies can help restore regularity to the menstrual cycle. This is always a difficult therapy, however, because the disorders are frequently quite complex, the hormones can have dangerous side effects, and most importantly, when used in excess, they can block the release of the body's own hormones, which is the opposite of the effect intended.

ACUPOINT TREATMENT

Acupoint therapy can often be quite successful in restoring absent or irregular periods. Through its systemic effect, it can take care of several combined problems and "synchronize" the menstrual periods on many levels.

TECHNIQUES TO USE

As the purpose is to trigger a flow, the stimulation has to be intense and deep or else done repeatedly until there are results. This will allow time to investigate the actual causes of the disorder, which may then be treated directly.

If the disorder is purely functional, the repetition of stimulation to the points in the morning and in the evening for three to five minutes at a time can restore the regular cycle.

The Points

The first point is located on the lower back, three finger-widths on either side of the spine, at the height level with the tops of the iliac crests.

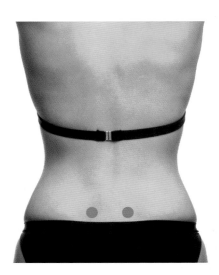 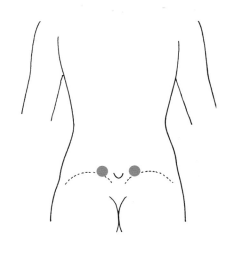

The Points (continued)

The second point is on the belly about a finger-width beneath the navel. The third is on the inside of the leg, a hand-width above the ankle in a small depression on the back edge of the tibia.

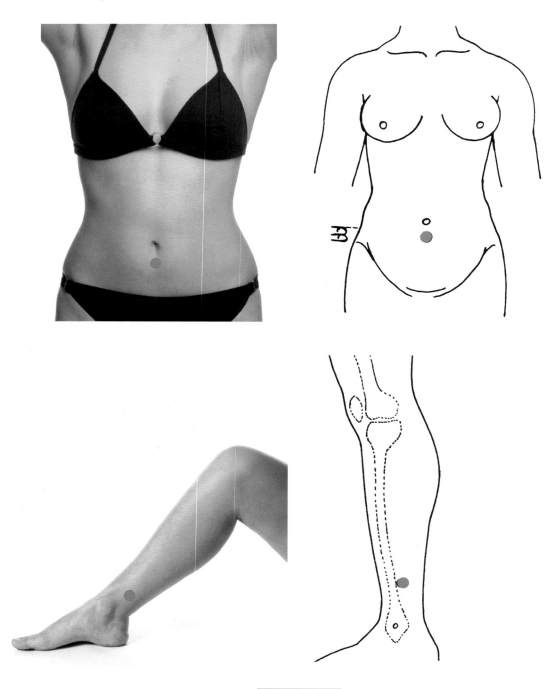

Menstrual Problems: Premenstrual Symptoms, Dysmenorrhea, and Irregular Periods

DYSMENORRHEA REFERS TO menstrual periods that are extremely painful. Therapeutically, this condition bears many similarities to the treatment of premenstrual symptoms and of irregular periods—those which come at irregular intervals, or are frequently longer or shorter than twenty-eight days.

Premenstrual symptoms may include emotional lability, swelling and pain in the breasts, weight gain, headaches, or digestive distress. A careful analysis of these elements can help pinpoint the exact cause of the problem.

The appearance of the menstrual blood can also be important: its color, whether deep or light red, and its consistency—whether it contains clots, membranes, and so forth—are also important indicators of underlying imbalances.

CAUSES

Problems affecting menstrual periods can originate in any level of the "sexual archi-tecture" depicted on page 246. The illnesses that can cause painful or irregular periods are the same, for the most part, as those that can bring about their complete absence.

STANDARD TREATMENT

Leaving aside the organic causes (cysts, tumors, and so on), menstrual disorders are generally treated with hormones, if they are treated at all. This is always a difficult therapy because it is double-edged. Hormones can have a curative effect, but they also pose a large risk of creating other problems. Most common of these is the fact that hormone-releasing glands will often cease to produce hormones when they are introduced into the body externally.

ACUPOINT TREATMENT

Acupuncture and acupressure, on the contrary, play a harmonizing role because they "regulate" the cycle: they do not over- or understimulate it. For this reason it is always worth trying, with the understanding, of course, that any physiological cause has been ruled out by the gynecologist.

TECHNIQUES TO USE

Here again the treatment will vary depending upon the underlying issue requiring treatment.

In the event of painful cramping, it is necessary to stimulate the points one week before the assumed date the period will begin. This stimulation should be for five minutes in the morning and again at night. If pain occurs with the period, stimulate the points for around twenty minutes until the suffering subsides.

If the cycles are irregular, or if the premenstrual phase brings uncomfortable symptoms, the points should be stimulated morning and night for fifteen minutes each over a three-week period, skipping over the week of the period itself.

The Principal Points

The points in common for all menstrual problems start with one point on the belly, halfway between the navel and the pubic bone; the second point is on the inside of the calf, a hand-width above the ankle in a small depression on the back edge of the tibia.

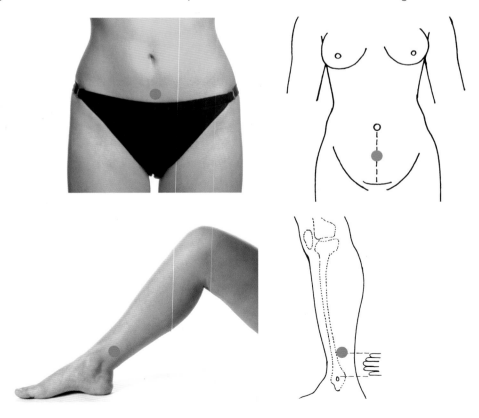

The Secondary Points

Add one or more of the secondary points below to address specific disorders.

For *pain* or *premenstrual symptoms:* one point is located on the upper edge of the pubic bone, two finger-widths from the median line; another is a hand-width beneath the crease of the knee on the outside of the leg. The point is in the small notch just below the head of the fibula.

For *abbreviated menstrual cycles* (less than twenty-eight days): one point is located on the lower thigh. To find it, cup the kneecap in your palm and lay your fingers on the thigh; your thumb will be on the point to stimulate.

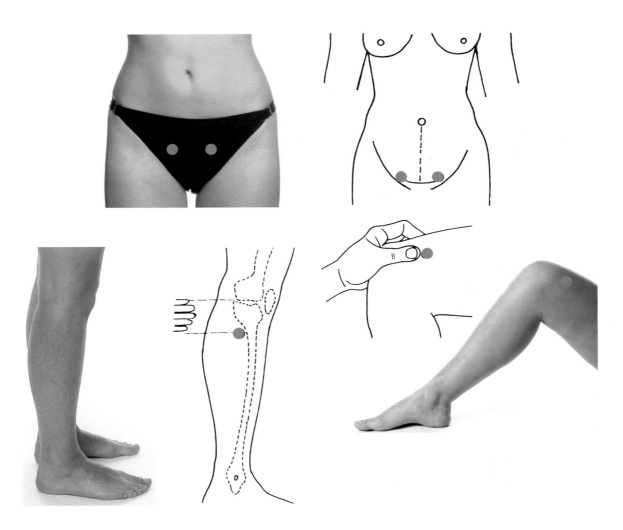

The Secondary Points (continued)

The second point can be found on the web between the first two toes. This point is also very good for premenstrual symptoms.

For *lengthened menstrual cycles:* one point is located on the inner edge of the foot, on the bone found at the halfway point; another is on the lower back, at the upper edge of the sacrum.

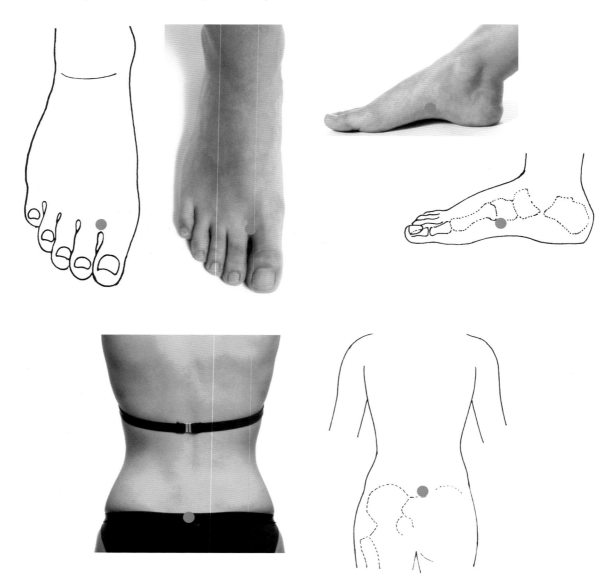

Uterine Hemorrhage

OF COURSE, BLOOD flow from the vagina is the major characteristic of menstruation and is quite a healthy event. But such flow would be considered abnormal under the following circumstances:

- If the menstrual flow is excessive in quantity or lasts too long (this hemorrhaging is called *menorrhagia*)
- If bleeding occurs outside the time of the menstrual period (known as *metrorrhagia*)
- If bleeding occurs before puberty or after menopause

Of course any hemorrhaging requires careful examination; severe blood loss can imperil a woman's life. In analyzing abnormal blood flow, it is important to know if the blood is red or black, and whether there are clots, fragments, or membranes in it. Is the odor normal or fetid? Is pus sometimes mixed with the blood? The accompanying symptoms must also be considered as hemorrhaging can sometimes be accompanied by pain, dizzy spells, vomiting, and so forth. All of this is of great importance in pinpointing the exact cause of the problem.

CAUSES

The causes are generally different for menorrhagia and metrorrhagia. The first is generally due to functional disorders or to a totally benign tumor like a fibroid.

Metrorrhagia can also be due to a disorder of functioning but it can also have a very serious cause such as tumors in the womb or elsewhere in close proximity, which can be malignant. Finally, general diseases such as infections or blood disorders may also be to blame.

STANDARD TREATMENT

The basic treatment, of course, depends upon the cause, and I will not go into great detail about those here. As a general rule, however, stopping the hemorrhage is a matter of complete urgency. For this purpose hemostatic drugs (meaning those that cause the blood to clot) are used, sometimes combined with hormones to force the fibers of the womb to contract.

ACUPOINT TREATMENT

Acupoint therapy is often quite effective for hemorrhages due to fibroids, as well as for other kinds of bleeding that do not arise from physiological lesions. Its innocuous nature and the speed with which it works make this therapy a valuable first line of defense, either by itself or in combination with another form of therapy.

TECHNIQUES TO USE

Treatment should be particularly intense when dealing with uterine hemorrhage; the most vigorous kinds of stimulation are called for here. This could be a prolonged massage of the different points in succession during which strong pressure is applied, or massage using a heated instrument (like a spoon, for example) taking care not to heat it so much that it burns the skin. In treating these kinds of cases, the practitioner most often uses electrical stimulation. Whatever form the stimulation takes, it should continue until the bleeding slows significantly or stops altogether.

To prevent the return of the hemorrhaging, stimulations of fifteen to twenty minutes should be performed two or three times a day.

The Principal Points

The first principal point is located on the lower outside corner of the toenail of the big toe; the second point is on the inner edge of the foot, behind the first joint of the toe.

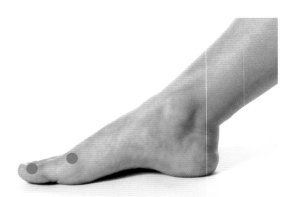
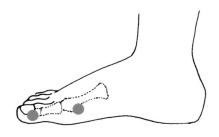

The Secondary Points

The first secondary point is in the center of the lower back, on the upper edge of the sacrum; the second point is located on the very top of the head at the intersection of the median line with a line going from one ear to the other.

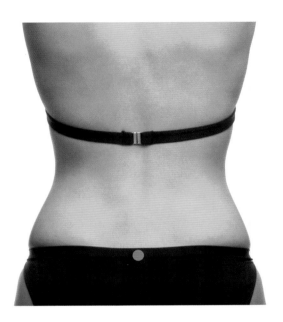

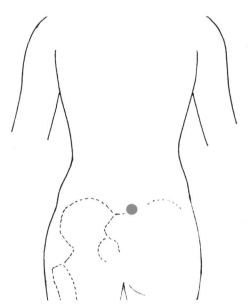

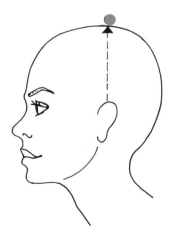

Uterine Prolapse

UTERINE PROLAPSE DESCRIBES the condition in which the uterus falls below its normal position in the pelvis. Initially the uterus will teeter backward before it starts descending. In this descent it can broadly relocate at the following different levels:

- to partially fill the vagina;
- to fill the vagina totally, in which case the cervix can be seen in the orifice of the vulva;
- though today this is quite exceptional, the uterus can emerge entirely and dangle between the legs.
- Finally, the womb's descent can drag down the neighboring organs, especially the bladder, whose function will be thereby disrupted.

SYMPTOMS AND FORMS

The descent of an organ like this causes a certain distinct discomfort—a kind of heaviness and burning—the sensation of having a heavy lump between the legs. Furthermore, the traction on the bladder in front and the constriction on the intestine behind will cause urinary problems and trouble evacuating the bowels. The severity of the condition will be evaluated depending on the scope of the organ's descent and its repercussions on the neighboring organs.

CAUSES

Uterine prolapse is due to weakness of the muscles and ligaments that normally support the uterus. The condition is most often due to difficult vaginal delivery, which can weaken the ligaments and muscles. Sometimes such weakened muscles will not cause a prolapse until menopause, when loss of muscle tone and reduced amounts of circulating estrogen further weaken the body's architecture.

STANDARD TREATMENT

When the descent of the womb is fairly advanced, only surgery is capable of fixing the situation—either by affixing the uterus within the pelvis or by removing it completely if the woman authorizes it. On the other hand, it is possible to intervene during the beginning stages and provide treatment to preserve the organ in its proper place. While keeping the organ in place with rubber diaphragms is rarely done anymore, Kegel exercises as described below can often improve the situation.

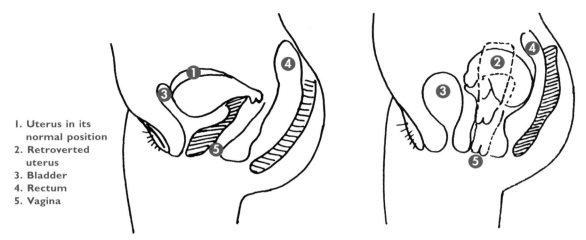

1. Uterus in its
   normal position
2. Retroverted
   uterus
3. Bladder
4. Rectum
5. Vagina

Depiction of uterine prolapse

ACUPOINT TREATMENT

Acupoint therapy can have its best effect during the initial stages of this disorder, combined, for example, with perineal physical therapy. On the other hand, once the descent is in an advanced state, surgery is the only option.

TECHNIQUES TO USE

Because this is a chronic disorder, it is necessary to stimulate these points for ten minutes in the morning and again at night, and combine this with exercises to strengthen the perineum. These Kegel exercises are quite well-known and quite simple: they involve clenching and releasing the pelvic floor muscles successively, several times in a row.

To find the pelvic floor muscles, practice stopping your stream of urine during urination. The muscles you use to do this are the pelvic floor muscles. In Kegel exercises, you clench and release these pelvic floor muscles repeatedly: clench and hold for one to four seconds, then release for an equal period of time. Repeat this cycle ten or more times, several times a day.

The Principal Points

The first principal point is located on the very top of the head at the intersection of the median line with a line going from one ear to the other.

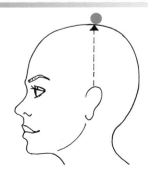

The Principal Points (continued)

The second point is on the front of the hips, two finger-widths above the iliac crest, the highest point of the pelvic bones.

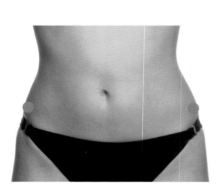

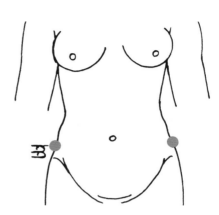

The Secondary Points

The first secondary point is on the top ridge of the pubic bone, two finger-widths on either side of the median line; the second is on the inside end of the knee crease.

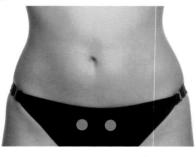

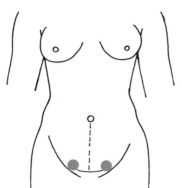

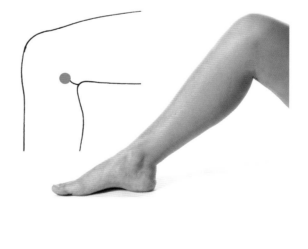

Leukorrhea

LEUKORRHEA IS TAKEN from the Greek term for "white discharge." It refers to any vaginal discharge that is not blood. Such discharges can be clear, white, yellowish, or greenish. They may be pasty or gelatinous, odorless or fetid. Important questions to ask about vaginal discharge include:

- At what point in the monthly cycle did these discharges occur? Are they occurring all the time or at only specific times during the menstrual cycle?
- What are the accompanying symptoms, if any? Pains, fever, contractions, and itching will all point to certain different causes.

CAUSES

Some cases of leukorrhea are perfectly normal: they occur at certain times during genital life—at ovulation, during the menstrual periods, or during pregnancy, for example. In these cases the discharges are generally very fluid and not profuse.

But if the discharge is yellow or green in color, this is an indication of infection, either by germs or a fungus.

Finally, discharges can be a symptom of a disease affecting the uterus or ovaries.

This is why a complete medical examination is always necessary.

STANDARD TREATMENT

Normal discharges should simply be left alone, but prurulent discharges should be treated by either a general medication or more often by disinfectant or antibiotic suppositories applied locally.

There are some antibiotics that are especially effective in fighting fungal infections.

ACUPOINT TREATMENT

Many of the new drugs unquestionably reduce leukorrhea symptoms, and thereby reduce the importance of acupoint stimulation for this condition, but the therapy can still offer reinforcement during treatment. For this reason, there is value in knowing what the points are.

TECHNIQUES TO USE

When abnormal discharge appears, massage the points vigorously for five minutes two to three times daily until it stops.

The Principal Point

The one principal point is located on the upper lip just beneath the nose.

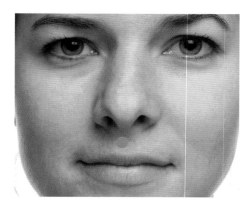
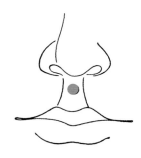

The Secondary Points

The first secondary point is on the top of the foot, in the web that joins the first two toes. The second point is beneath the knee on the inside of the leg, in the notch just below the head of the tibia bone.

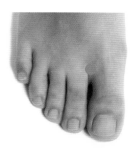
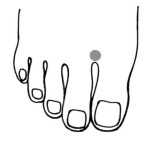
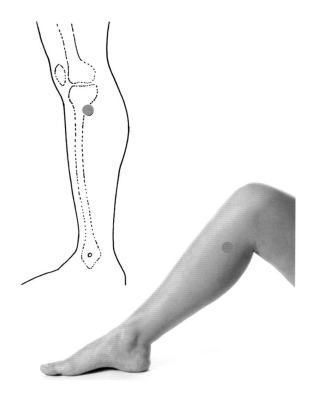

PART TWELVE

Miscellaneous

Fatigue

IS THERE ANY symptom more widespread than fatigue? Most of us hear expressions of exhaustion falling from the mouths of our contemporaries almost daily. Does this mean they are excessively exerting themselves physically? Hardly, it is rather the opposite.

There are actually two kinds of fatigue. One is the kind generated by athletic activity, for example what is felt at the end of a sporting event. The other is that of the modern worker who spends all day in an office, constantly badgered by visitors and telephone calls, traffic delays and everyday frustrations. This second is the most widespread form—so-called nervous fatigue—but the experiences are similar for both kinds.

In both cases, the points depicted here are particularly effective, whether the original cause of fatigue was physical exertion, nervous pressure, growing pains, or old age.

Massage these points for two to three minutes in succession. After this time, you will already be feeling better. Repeat the stimulation two or three times a day to drive away that unpleasant sense of exhaustion.

The Points

The first important point for fatigue is located two finger-widths below the navel on the median line.

The second point can be found on the outside of the leg. This is how to find it: It is three finger-widths beneath the tip of the kneecap, and two finger-widths behind the crest of the tibia. (This is the larger leg bone, which runs down the front of the leg.) In any event, do not be worried if this point is hard to pinpoint. It will react to any pressure on this area of the skin.

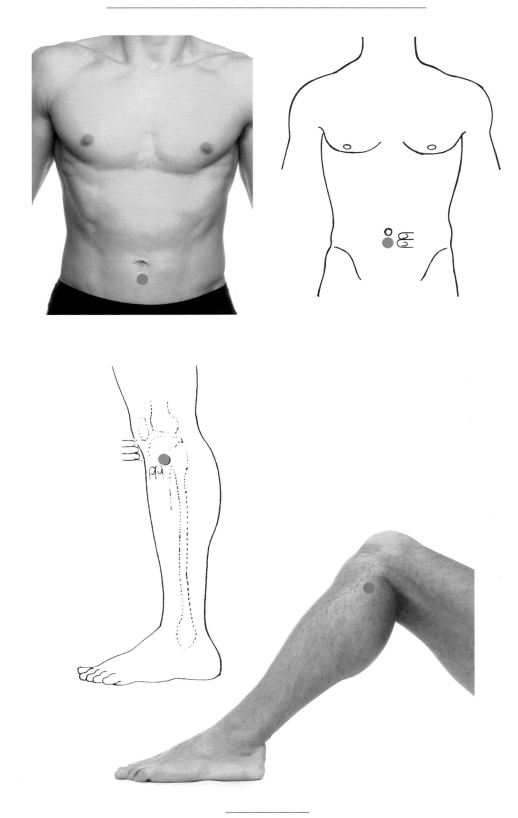

Insomnia

SLEEP IS LIKE a very complicated and very delicate piece of machinery, whose mysteries researchers are barely beginning to decipher.

What we do know presently is that there are several kinds of sleep that follow each other in alternation during the course of the night. There is non-REM sleep, characterized by four stages of varying depths of sleep, and there is REM sleep, during which the sleeper dreams.

Aren't dreams the translation of our deepest hopes and needs and tendencies? More importantly, dreams provide the means of integrating within ourselves what we have acquired over the day. They therefore play an enormous role in our mental equilibrium.

Just as there are two basic kinds of sleep there are also two different kinds of insomnia. One is the insomnia that keeps people awake at the beginning of the night and the other is an insomnia that has a tendency to come on closer to the dawn. This form seems more connected to stress, anxiety, and depression.

However, whichever of the two kinds of insomnia a person may be experiencing, these points work on both varieties.

Massage both points slowly and deeply in succession and sleep will come without any need to resort to chemical drugs.

The Points

The principal point is located on the second toe, at the lower corner of the toenail on the side nearest the little toe.

A secondary point is on the inside of the foot at the base of the big toe.

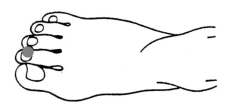

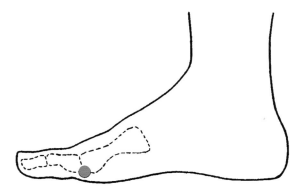

Stage Fright

HOW MANY BUDDING speaking and acting careers, how many students' aspirations, have been broken by this disorder that locks up the throat, dries out the mouth, and turns the legs to water?

This is why it is so valuable to have a point that is so easy to reach and fairly discreet, one that can if not banish stage fright entirely, reduce it considerably. It is equally helpful for calming high emotion and moral outrage.

This point is literally right at hand. It can be found on the right side of the chest, four finger-widths beneath the collarbone, directly above the nipple.

This point can be massaged lengthily—and discreetly, as if you were scratching yourself, for example—until you are feeling calm again.

The Point

The point is located on the right side of the chest, four finger-widths below the clavicle (collar-bone).

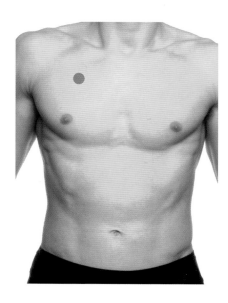
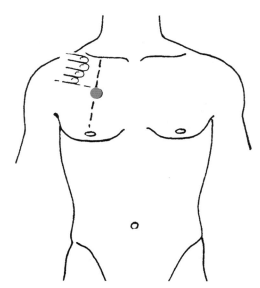

Stings or Bites
from Poisonous Animals

TO PREPARE ADEQUATELY for the possibility of poisoning by insect or animal, we must first think about the many venomous creatures that fly, crawl, swim, and otherwise inopportunely cross our paths. Naturally, the degree of damage they can cause us varies enormously from a simple irritant to a life-threatening injury.

The severity of the consequences depends on three things:

- First, of course, is the nature and quantity of the venom introduced into the body. There is obviously nothing similar between the simple irritant of a mosquito's bite and the toxic matter poured into our bodies by the venom glands of a viper!

- But the outcome also depends on the general health of the victim. If we are in poor health, exhausted, and already more sensitive to a particular venom because of an allergy or an earlier attack, even a modest injection can have tragic results.

This is the case with bee and wasp stings in particular. For some people these stings will be followed only by a smarting pain that is annoying but tolerable. Others, though, will experience immediate shock, with the possible loss of consciousness, cardiac problems, and, in the most serious cases, death.

- Finally, the place where a person is stung is also significant. Even for a person who has no particular sensitivity to stings, a sting in the throat by an inopportunely swallowed wasp will trigger a huge swelling of the mucous membranes that can obstruct the respiratory tract.

Let's take a quick look at what kind of venomous animals we need to fear. In Europe, the different species of vipers pose the gravest risk; in the United States there are only four kinds of poisonous snakes, most of which are more to be dreaded in the southern reaches of the country. These are rattlesnakes, copperheads, water moccasins, and coral snakes—the deadliest of this group—whose bite is often fatal.

Among insects the most worrisome are bees (including bumblebees), wasps, and yellow jackets. Dozens of deaths, if not more, can be attributed to insect stings every year in Europe and North America. Horseflies and mosquitoes are simply irritating (except in the event of malaria, which is spread by mosquitoes in the tropics and more recently,

West Nile Virus, which can be dangerous to the elderly and infirm). There are then fleas, bedbugs, and ticks in particular, who are responsible for the spread of Lyme disease, Rocky Mountain spotted fever, and several other dangerous illnesses. There are also a few spiders to worry about, including the black widow, the brown recluse, and some species of tarantula, and finally, chiggers.

Among sea creatures we have stingrays and weever fish, among others. Unwary bathers can be stung, which causes a generally brief sensation of intense pain and some swelling. Finally, jellyfish are becoming increasingly common in the waters and on the beach, and their touch can trigger a burning and irritating rash, swelling, and tissue death. Some species can be fatal.

STANDARD TREATMENT

The treatments are quite varied—as one might imagine—according to the nature and seriousness of the poison.

Calming creams and lotions generally are enough for mosquito bites, while snakebite has to be treated at the site of the incident or at the hospital by powerful drugs like adrenalin, cortisone, and so forth. For some kinds of snakebite—like that of the coral snake—the antivenin vaccines are the only successful treatment.

Finally, treatments to counter the sensitivity to wasp and bee venom are used before the advent of summer for those individuals at risk. Homeopathic treatment is particularly recommended in this instance.

But no matter how inconsequential or serous the venom, a certain number of actions need to be performed or avoided. First, immediately following the bite or sting, do not apply pressure above the wound in the hope of causing the venom to exit; that will simply ensure that it spreads through the body much more thoroughly. Next, place a burning object as close as possible to the bite as many venoms are, in fact, destroyed by heat. In antiquity, red-hot irons were applied to snakebites, but a simple lit cigarette can spoil up to three quarts of injected venom. Finally, stimulate two acupuncture points with which the Chinese are extremely familiar (death from snakebite is quite common in there).

ACUPOINT TREATMENT

Massage the points slowly for a long time or, even better, if you have an electrical stimulator at hand, use that.

The Points

The first point to stimulate is located on the outside of the arm. With the arm bent, it is a finger-width above the crease of the elbow, against the bone.

The second point is midway between the knee and ankle on the outside of the leg, just against the bone.

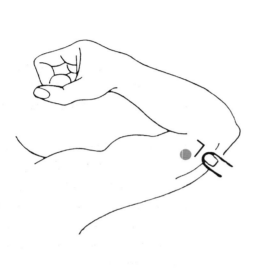

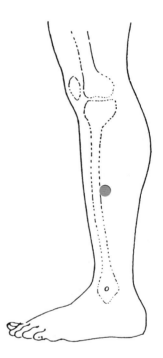

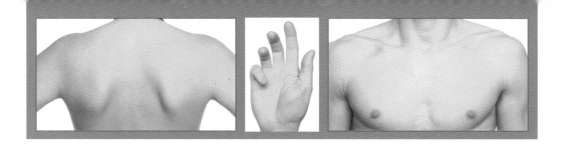

Conclusion

OVER THE COURSE of this book, I have made an effort to describe how Chinese acupoints can be used in the treatment of numerous diseases and disorders. A little focus is all it takes to pinpoint the location of the points described in this book, but the list of useful points included here is by no means exhaustive; there are many, many others.

The long history and diverse nature of Chinese medicine have bequeathed to us a style of medicine that provides dozens, if not hundreds, of approaches to any given symptom. Most practitioners will have their favorite points or sets of points for particular ailments; many of these will have been passed down from teacher to student for generations. Still others will be modern points, "discovered" by systematic research or lucky chance.

Treatments using points other than the ones described in this book—alone or in combination with other therapies—can also produce excellent results. If you find yourself interested in this style of medicine, I invite you to seek out one of the many available workshops and seminars that give more explicit instruction in acupoint locations and therapies.

That this method may provide relief without causing any harm is this author's dearest wish!

Index

Page numbers in *italics* represent illustrations.

BOOKS OF RELATED INTEREST

The Acupressure Atlas
by Bernard C. Kolster, M.D.,
and Astrid Waskowiak, M.D.

The Reflexology Atlas
by Bernard C. Kolster, M.D.,
and Astrid Waskowiak, M.D.

Acupressure Taping
The Practice of Acutaping for Chronic Pain and Injuries
by Hans-Ulrich Hecker, M.D., and Kay Liebchen, M.D.

Trigger Point Therapy for Myofascial Pain
The Practice of Informed Touch
by Donna Finando, L.Ac., L.M.T.,
and Steven Finando, Ph.D., L.Ac.

Trigger Point Self-Care Manual
For Pain-Free Movement
by Donna Finando, L.Ac., L.M.T.

Acupressure Techniques
A Self-Help Guide
by Julian Kenyon, M.D.

Facial Reflexology
A Self-Care Manual
by Marie-France Muller, M.D., N.D., Ph.D.

Reflex Zone Therapy of the Feet
A Comprehensive Guide for Health Professionals
by Hanne Marquardt

INNER TRADITIONS • BEAR & COMPANY
P.O. Box 388
Rochester, VT 05767
1-800-246-8648
www.InnerTraditions.com

Or contact your local bookseller